Mary Carolan

Doing it Properly

Transition to motherhood for first-time mothers 35 years and above

LAP LAMBERT Academic Publishing

Impressum/Imprint (nur für Deutschland/ only for Germany)

Bibliografische Information der Deutschen Nationalbibliothek: Die Deutsche Nationalbibliothek verzeichnet diese Publikation in der Deutschen Nationalbibliografie; detaillierte bibliografische Daten sind im Internet über http://dnb.d-nb.de abrufbar.

Alle in diesem Buch genannten Marken und Produktnamen unterliegen warenzeichen-, marken- oder patentrechtlichem Schutz bzw. sind Warenzeichen oder eingetragene Warenzeichen der jeweiligen Inhaber. Die Wiedergabe von Marken, Produktnamen, Gebrauchsnamen, Handelsnamen, Warenbezeichnungen u.s.w. in diesem Werk berechtigt auch ohne besondere Kennzeichnung nicht zu der Annahme, dass solche Namen im Sinne der Warenzeichen- und Markenschutzgesetzgebung als frei zu betrachten wären und daher von jedermann benutzt werden dürften.

Coverbild: www.ingimage.com

Verlag: LAP LAMBERT Academic Publishing AG & Co. KG
Dudweiler Landstr. 99, 66123 Saarbrücken, Deutschland
Telefon +49 681 3720-310, Telefax +49 681 3720-3109
Email: info@lap-publishing.com

Herstellung in Deutschland:
Schaltungsdienst Lange o.H.G., Berlin
Books on Demand GmbH, Norderstedt
Reha GmbH, Saarbrücken
Amazon Distribution GmbH, Leipzig
ISBN: 978-3-8383-7599-1

Imprint (only for USA, GB)

Bibliographic information published by the Deutsche Nationalbibliothek: The Deutsche Nationalbibliothek lists this publication in the Deutsche Nationalbibliografie; detailed bibliographic data are available in the Internet at http://dnb.d-nb.de.

Any brand names and product names mentioned in this book are subject to trademark, brand or patent protection and are trademarks or registered trademarks of their respective holders. The use of brand names, product names, common names, trade names, product descriptions etc. even without a particular marking in this works is in no way to be construed to mean that such names may be regarded as unrestricted in respect of trademark and brand protection legislation and could thus be used by anyone.

Cover image: www.ingimage.com

Publisher: LAP LAMBERT Academic Publishing AG & Co. KG
Dudweiler Landstr. 99, 66123 Saarbrücken, Germany
Phone +49 681 3720-310, Fax +49 681 3720-3109
Email: info@lap-publishing.com

Printed in the U.S.A.
Printed in the U.K. by (see last page)
ISBN: 978-3-8383-7599-1

3

Acknowledgements

It is with great appreciation that I would like to thank my children, Emer, Aoife and Andrew, each of whom has contributed positively to this work. Thank you all for your patience and forbearance when I have often been unavailable to you. I would particularly like to thank Professor Sioban Nelson who has been a great source of inspiration and intellectual stimulation for me. Thanks also to my midwifery colleagues at Jessie MacPherson Hospital who have unanimously assisted and encouraged my efforts. Special thanks to Di Sexton, Ellice McLaren, Maggie Brougham and Chris Crossbie for proofreading and advice. Finally, and most importantly, I would like to acknowledge the mothers of this study, without whom this research could not have taken place.

CHAPTER 1
INTRODUCTION

This work is concerned with the experiences of contemporary first mothering for women over 35 years, a new social category of mothers. My interest in this area has developed over many years of midwifery practice, during which I have seen marked demographic changes in parturition[1] trends. In the mid '80s when I was a primigravida, the term 'elderly primigravida' related to first-time mothers greater than 25 yrs. Medical circles were full of dire warnings about the dangers of delaying parturition beyond this juncture. The bones of the pelvis become rigid and inflexible after this time announced one of the midwifery textbooks of the day, making natural childbirth more difficult (Myles, 1985). By the 1990s the trend for later commencement of parturition was well established, but curiously devoid of public censure, though medically the practice of older childbearing was viewed as fraught with danger, related principally to infant mortality and morbidity (Cnattingius, Forman, Berendes & Isotalo, 1992; Peipert & Bracken, 1993).

In my place of work, a private hospital affiliated with a tertiary level public hospital, I have become aware of a gradual change in client profile to include an increasing proportion of older first-time mothers who are predominantly career women. These women approach mothering differently than average-aged or less high achieving women and seem to 'manage' this new stage as they would any major project, by reading all the available information and formulating a plan. It was not uncommon to come upon just such a woman breastfeeding, guided by a diagram in a book. Several times I have seen an older primipara detach a correctly positioned infant, explaining that his/her mouth didn't resemble the diagram. When asked how the attachment felt, or if it was painful, the mother would not have taken this into consideration. I found it difficult to comprehend that a woman could be so removed from the experience of breastfeeding her infant.

Then my sister Elizabeth, an established career woman, aged 39 years, 'HAD A BABY' at a considerably later time than our siblings. Our mother, herself a veteran of 10 children, described Elizabeth's pregnancy as 'more trouble than all of you together'. This was in spite of Elizabeth having a normal pregnancy and having previously been exposed to children through growing up in a large family, though as a younger member of the family she may have had a limited memory of this

---

[1] childbearing

experience. In her quest for information, Elizabeth had attended no fewer than four workshops and two complete sets of prenatal education classes and had read as many as 30 books on 'mothering'. She had also read extensively on cognitive stimulation in the newborn and, when asked by her siblings why she was making such a fuss, her reply was that she just wanted to 'do it properly'. This phrase 'doing it properly' seemed to me to encapsulate the experiences of first-time mothers older than 35 that I commonly met with in my own clinical practice, so much so, that I pondered on the differences displayed by such women and the social antecedents informing this approach.

For myself, a midwife, I was confused by the paradox this situation offered. Many older primiparae are established career or business women (Berkowitz, Shoran, Lapinski & Berkowitz, 1993; Ozer, 1995; Ventura, 1989) with a prior history of capability, and it seemed strange that they might be defeated by mothering. I felt certain that the social context of these women's lives had some bearing on their experiences. To that end, I was keen to investigate the experience of first mothering for women over 35 years of age.

In general, later first mothering appears to be problematic and there is considerable anecdotal evidence to suggest that transition to motherhood among 'elderly primigravidae'[2] is fraught with difficulty. In particular, these difficulties are said to include heightened anxiety (Nicholson, 1998) and a postulated increased incidence of postnatal depression[3]. Greater attendance at mother and baby units is also noted (Fisher, Feekery, Amir & Sneddon, 2002). Additionally, from my clinical midwifery practice, I am aware of nursing perceptions of older primiparae as 'difficult' and 'needy' in terms of consuming nursing time and resources. Many midwifery, medical and nursing staff describe caring for this group of women as stressful and challenging, labelling the mothers 'hopeless', 'past it' and as 'deliberately making it [mothering] difficult'. This understanding is similar to that expressed by Dobrzykowski (1998), who found that nursing staff viewed older first-time mothers as "difficult to work with, hysterical and psychologically challenging" (p. 4).

This study was thus concerned with the experience of later first mothering. Specifically, it sought to discover if this group of mothers had special needs or concerns during their transition to motherhood. Ultimately, it was hoped that the knowledge gained during this research endeavour would add to the

---

[2] In 1958 the council of the International Federation of Gynecologists & Obstetricians recommended that a primigravida aged 35 years or more be labeled an "elderly primigravida" (Barkan & Bracken, 1987). In general, 35 years appears to have become accepted as the cut-off point for increased pregnancy risks. Increased prenatal screening such as amniocentesis for chromosomal abnormalities is routinely offered for pregnant women over 35 years of age.

[3] Maternal depression following birth commonly described as postnatal depression in Australia and as postpartum depression in the U.S.A.

8

scant body of literature addressing older first-mothering and inform strategies to better meet the specific needs of this group of otherwise healthy mothers.

In this chapter, a brief examination of changing birth demographics is attended, followed by an exploration of the emergence of primigravidae over 35 as a social phenomenon. It is my contention that an understanding of the emergence of the 'elderly primigravida' and accompanying social expectations is fundamental to any appreciation of the inherent difficulties of maternal role transition for these women. Issues of transition to motherhood for primiparae over 35 are then discussed together with the research question and aims of the current study. In the final section of this chapter, an outline of the structure of the work is presented.

Introduction

Later childbearing is an increasingly common trend in advanced industrial nations and this trend has been steadily growing for more than two decades. Contributing factors include changing societal values, decreasing family sizes and greater social acceptance of later commencement of childbearing. Other suggested factors are increasing female workforce participation and higher education. Current social discourses dictate that a woman can 'have it all', that is, fulfilling career, economic opportunity, satisfying social life, sexual relationship and children (Hoffnung 1995). However, we will see that these social expectations also complicate the experience of childbearing for contemporary women, many of whom now take up mothering in the context of career commitments and at an older age than previous generations. In order to have an understanding of whence these women have come socially, it is important to first consider demographic and social changes of the last few decades, as follows.

Demographic shifts in birthing trends

Birthing trends in advanced industrial nations have changed remarkably over the past few decades, demonstrating: declining birth-rates; increasing median age of childbearing and reducing teen birth-rates (Australian Bureau of Statistics [ABS], 2000, 2003a; Australian Institute of Health and Welfare [AIHW], 2000; U.K. National Statistics, 2001; U.S. Center for Disease Control and Prevention [U.S. National Vital Statistic reports], 2001a, 2001b) though the rate of decline among teen births varies. In Britain and the U.S.A., the percentage of teen births remains strikingly higher than Australian rates (ABS, 2000).

For the purpose of locating changing patterns of childbearing internationally, birthing trends in Australia, the U.S.A. and Britain are briefly reviewed. These countries are chosen as representative of westernised nations[4], wherein the phenomenon of elderly primiparity is especially marked. As the current study is located in Australia, emphasis is placed on Australian birthing trends.

Historical overview

Birthing trends for Australia, the United States and Britain show strikingly parallel fluctuations over the last century, responding to similar social, economic and political influences. The two world wars impacted significantly on the number of births occurring in each of these countries, as their young men went off to war and were absent sometimes for several years. Significant population increases (baby booms) marked the years following the world wars. For example, in 1920, Britain registered 1.1 million births, the highest number for any year in the 20th century (U.K. National Statistics, 2001). Rates were similarly high in Australia (ABS, 2000) and in the U.S.A. (U.S. National Vital Statistic reports 2001a) during the 1920s. These upward trends continued for approximately ten years when a significant downturn occurred (ABS, 2000; U.K. National Statistics, 2001; U.S. National Vital Statistics reports 2001a) related to the depressed economic climate of the 1930s. This downward trend continued until the mid 1940s as low birth rates occurred throughout WWII years (1939-1945).

Immediately following WWII, Australia, the U.S.A. and Britain all experienced baby booms that continued until the late 1950s/1960s. These population peaks were undoubtedly influenced by the socio-political imperatives of the day and a sense of urgency to replace lives lost during the war years. Post war economic prosperity also most likely contributed. In addition to fluctuations in fertility rate, the demographics of giving birth have changed considerably since the 1960s, particularly in regard to increasing maternal age and those changes are now considered.

The 'greying' of the maternal population

In Australia, the median age of all mothers has risen to 30.2 years in 2002, from just 26.3 years in 1978 (ABS, 2000; ABS, 2003a; AIHW, 2000). In Britain, median age for giving birth has also increased steadily, from 23.9 years in 1968 to 28.9 in 1998, while in the U.S.A., median age at childbearing has risen from approximately 22.0 years in 1972 to 24.5 years in 1999 (U.S. National Vital Statistics Report. Vol. 49, No. 4, 2001) though it remains considerably lower than the Australian and British figures, most likely related to comparatively higher U.S. teen birth rates. Together with increasing median age for giving birth, other new birthing trends have emerged in the past two decades. These

---

[4] Advanced industrial nations of the first world

trends include postponement of first births and the gradual 'greying' of the maternal population, discussed as follows.

The emergence of the elderly primipara / a new social phenomenon

The 'greying' of the maternal population is an increasingly prevalent trend in the advanced industrial world and first-time mothers make up an increasing percentage of this group. From this point, the discussion of birth demographics relates primarily to Australian trends, in line with the intent of this study. At present, the birth rate for women aged over 35 years is growing faster than for any other age group in Australia as demonstrated in the graph below (2.2 ABS, 2003a, p. 9). In 2002, 18.2% of Australian mothers were aged more than 35 years (ABS, 2003a) compared to less than half that number in 1979 (ABS, 2000).

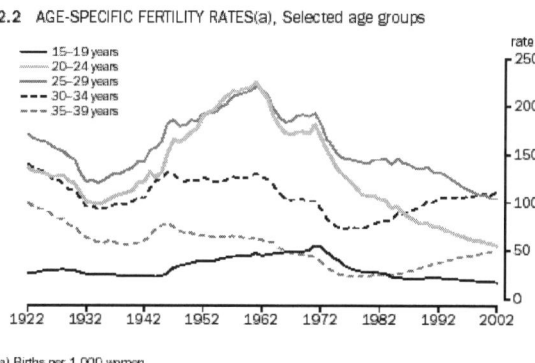

2.2 AGE-SPECIFIC FERTILITY RATES(a), Selected age groups

- 15–19 years
- 20–24 years
- 25–29 years
- 30–34 years
- 35–39 years

(a) Births per 1,000 women.

(ABS 2003a p.9)

Figures for first births among older mothers are also significant and increasing (AIHW, 2000) and, although older childbearing in itself is not new, current trends are markedly different than previously. Previously, older childbearing tended to be most common among the lower social echelons (Wildschut, 1999), representing multigravid women[5] who had commenced childbearing several years earlier. Older primiparity[6] was a relatively unusual event and was most commonly related to late marriages,

---

[5] women who have had more than 1 pregnancy

[6] first mothering

infertility (Harker & Thorpe, 1992) and, occasionally, deliberate choice in times of hardship, as during the depression years of the 1930s (ABS, 2000).

Today increasing numbers of women electively delay parturition until older than 35 years in pursuit of career / educational opportunities, and this represents a new social phenomenon. Throughout westernised nations this cohort tends to represent a considerably different social group from older mothers of two to three decades ago. Now, although not homogeneous, this cohort tends to consist of well-educated women (Berryman, Thorpe & Windridge, 1999; Stark, 1997) participating in highly paid employment, many of whom are professionals, for example, lawyers, doctors and accountants (Berkowitz et al., 1993; Berryman et al., 1999; Ozer, 1995). As such, these women are likely to be financially secure (Cunningham & Leveno, 1995), to pursue healthy lifestyle choices (Berryman et al., 1999), to eat a balanced diet and to abstain from smoking (Berryman et al., 1999; Najman, Lanyon, Andersen, Williams, Bor & O'Callaghan, 1998; Ventura, 1989). Higher maternal education is also commonly associated with increased health awareness and greater use of health care facilities (Morrison, Najman, Williams, Keeping & Anderson, 1989; Raum, Arabin, Schlaud, Walter & Schwartz, 2001; Richman, Miller & LeVine, 1992).

Overall, as part of a predominantly healthy and well-educated cohort, this group of mothers is likely to experience significantly lower risk than a group of contemporaries of 20–40 years ago, who were often grand multiparae[7]. The associated risks of grand multiparity, including: anaemia; malpresentation of the fetus; macrosomic[8] infants; obstetric haemorrhage (Bennett & Brown, 1999; Dildy et al., 1996; Wildschut, 1999) and socio-economic disadvantage (Wall, Khoshnood, Singh, Hsieh & Lee, 1998; Wildschut, 1999) are well known and have informed much of the persisting medical opinion associated with advanced maternal age. In the following section, this association of medical 'risk' and older maternity is discussed.

Risk / clinical issues

Medical research identifies the older mother as 'at risk' for a range of complications and this risk perception also informs the subsequent care these women receive. In focusing predominantly on medical risk, pregnant women over 35 are often labelled 'high risk' once they enter the healthcare system and may have restrictions placed on care options and their choice of birth venue. Indeed, the older mother is frequently exposed to increased pregnancy surveillance (Berryman et al., 1999;

---

[7] women who have had more than 5 children
[8] large infant weighing more than 4.0kg, often related to maternal diabetes

Windridge & Berryman, 1996) and will most probably be offered additional screening tests (Muggli & Halliday, 2003), which in turn may fuel maternal angst. It is my contention, based on my midwifery experience, that this emphasis on 'risk' may carry serious ramifications for the woman's confidence in her ability to carry her pregnancy to term and to successfully give birth to her baby.

Other issues for this group include declining fertility and concomitant emotional issues. In general, natural pregnancy after 39 years of age is considered to be rare and after 44 years is considered exceptional (Cohen & Sauer, 1998) though many contemporary women consider that they can rely on getting pregnant well into their forties (Burrage, 1998; Hewlett, 2002b). The discovery of age-related fertility decline often occurs only after a decision to have a baby has been reached (Hewlett, 2002a). Although increasingly sophisticated technology presents fertility options to women who might not otherwise have had children, the process may be far from unproblematic, as we shall see in later chapters. In addition to medical risk perception, social mores also impact on maternal experience for this group of women, as follows.

Older mothering / timing of pregnancy / mixed messages

Changing social patterns contribute to trends of later childbearing but also impact on maternal experiences for contemporary women. The taking on of maternal identity is generally understood to be complex and multi-dimensional but, for first-time mothers over 35, the experience appears to be compounded by other factors such as limited social support and confusing expectations. Older timing mothers are in general, considered less likely to live close to family supports than younger mothers (Ambler Walter, 1986; Cook, 1993; Reece, 1995) and may also have fewer social networks. Many such mothers have little or no experience of young children and may feel out of time with peers. Indeed, according to Daniels and Weingarten (1982), every era or generation has an "implicit consensus about the right time" to become a parent, that is contingent on social mores (p. 13). In contemporary Australia, the 'right' time to have a first baby is approximately 28-30 years, similar to the median age of childbearing (ABS, 2003a). Although there is some room for variation, most health professionals consider maternity when aged over 35 years to be risky (Anderson, Wohlfahrt, Christens, Olsen & Melbye, 2000; Cnattingius et al., 1992; Fretts, 2001). Women choosing to delay childbearing beyond this juncture may feel 'out of time' with regard to social norms (Dobrzykowski & Stern, 2003; Neurgarten & Datan, 1973; Rossi, 1980) and contemporaries may be the mothers of teenagers at the same time as the older primipara is the mother of an infant.

Additionally, many women now mother whilst continuing with career plans and, indeed, women are expected to work, both to contribute to family finances and for personal fulfilment (Filene, 1998). Nonetheless, social expectations around mothering and employment are confusing and paradoxical and women are also expected to mother as a fulfilling and essential female role (Thurer, 1994). As pro-natalistic societies, much of the advanced industrial world advocates the importance of the family and the central position of the child within the family. Decreasing birth rates add to the social significance of the individual child and also to the work of raising him/her. However, despite apparent strong social approval, mothering attracts less social value than employment. A further difficulty presents for contemporary women who have been socialised through their school and work experiences to value independence and individuality (Hoffnung, 1995, p. 166). Social expectations around mothering confusingly dictate sacrificial maternal behaviours and place the infant's needs ahead of the mother's, which is in contrast to social values for modern women. Additionally, despite growing trends of female employment, motherhood and personal ambition are largely seen as opposing forces (Thurer, 1994), and it is this tension that is central to the conundrum of mothering / womanly identity for modern women. These difficulties are experienced by new mothers of all ages but seem to be heightened among women used to agency and autonomy in the public sphere. Older mothers, who may have exercised authority in their lives and have worked for a considerably longer time than their younger counterparts, may thus be particularly affected. For these women, transition to motherhood is frequently associated with maladjustment and difficulty, as discussed in the following section.

Transition issues

Anecdotal evidence suggests that older first-time mothers experience significant distress and anxiety around transition to motherhood, which is unrelated or out of proportion to medical risks or potential complications. In general, the psychosocial vulnerability of older mothers is well known (Nicholson, 1998) and high levels of anxiety, unrelated to health issues, are considered to be common for this group. Postnatal depression (PND), a serious condition affecting approximately 10% of new mothers (Bewley, 1999; Green, 1998; Warner, Appleby, Whitton & Faragher, 1996) and associated with a significant cost to the community in terms of maternal morbidity, poorer infant attachment and strained family relationships (Brown, Lumley, Small & Astbury, 1994), is thought to be more prevalent among older first-time mothers. Suggested predisposing factors for this serious condition are maternal age (Stowe & Nemeroff, 1995), psychological distress or anxiety during pregnancy (Forman, Videbech, Hedegaard, Salvig & Secher, 2000; Kurstjens & Wolke, 2001; Stowe & Nemeroff, 1995), socio-professional difficulties (Righetti-Veltema, Conne-Perreard, Bousquet & Manzano, 1998) and "dyadic discord accentuated by traditional sex role expectations" (Steinberg & Bellavance, 1999, p. 209), meaning traditional division of labour at home. Individual personality traits have also been implicated (Bewley, 1999) and there is some suggestion that older first-time mothers exhibit greater personal autonomy than their younger counterparts and also that this trait may negatively affect their transition to motherhood (Windridge & Berryman, 1999).

However, despite a postulated link between older primiparity and higher than usual levels of anxiety (Steinberg & Bellavance, 1999; Stowe & Nemeroff, 1995; Windridge & Berryman, 1999) and prominent suggestions of higher levels of maladjustment and postnatal depression, when reviewing the literature it becomes clear that little is known about the experiences of mothering for first-time mothers over 35 years. Specifically, the socio-political and cultural antecedents of maternal adjustment are not well attended (Rogan, Schmied, Barclay, Everitt & Wyllie, 1997) and few studies have concentrated on the social context in which new mothering occurs, particularly for primiparae over 35. This dearth gives rise to the current research question.

Problem statement / research question

The increasing phenomenon of older maternity, particularly career-orientated middle-class postponers, raises a number of interesting questions. For instance, are older mothers more at risk, in terms of psychological well being in pregnancy and early motherhood? If so, what implications does this carry for maternal and infant health? Do older primiparous mothers, often with many years of career investment, find it more difficult to adjust to maternity? Does this group of mothers suffer from increased incidences of maternal maladjustment and postnatal depression, as frequently expected? Does maternal maturity have any positive effects for women having infants later than average?

Most importantly, the social context of mothering for these women is an area that has received scant attention to date, although it is clear that changing life trajectories and employment impact significantly on the experiences of contemporary mothers.

Additionally, as the age of childbearing women in Australia and, indeed, globally, continues to rise and the health dollar continues to shrink, implications for the health and well being of the older mother and her infant assumes previously unknown proportions. In the current climate of fiscal austerity, which is characterised by ever earlier discharge from hospital following birth and fewer maternal and child health services, it becomes increasingly important that health professionals learn as much as possible about the needs and concerns of this group of women to better assist them in their transition to motherhood. This study sought to address the following question primarily:

1. What is the experience of first mothering for women over 35 years?

A second and lesser question related to midwifery and maternal and child health nurses' views of older primiparae. In particular, this second question sought to address the clinical issues identified by health professionals as related specifically to first maternity older than 35 years.

Data was collected in the following way. In-depth interviewing of mothers occurred over three junctures and the interviews are fully described in chapter 3. Three focus groups of midwives and maternal and child health nurses [M&CHNs][9] were also conducted in a bid to provide background information and to help frame the research question. Focus group data and discussion is presented in appendix C.

Finally, because this work is primarily concerned with postpartum experience and adjustment, limited attention is accorded to pregnancy, per se, other than as a staging for later maternal experience. Similiarly, fathers and paternal experience are notably absent. The theoretical framework of this work, which is explored in greater detail in the

following chapter, draws on both post-structural and feminist theories. Within this view, a particular valuing of women's accounts is possible and the individual is seen as being shaped by the social discourses of the day. It is the premise of this work that social context powerfully affects women's mothering experiences.

Structure of the work

This introduction has provided an historical overview of demographic shifts in childbearing trends, particularly trends of later childbearing and the emergence of the older primipara. A limited understanding of the social context of mothering for these women is identified. Chapter 2 presents a discussion of the changing social context of contemporary women's lives and emphasis is accorded to the growing selfhood of modern women. Here the author uses a particular narrative style and contrasts

---

[9] In Victoria, Australia, mothers and infants are cared for in Maternal and Child Health Centres following discharge from hospital. Mothers attend with their infants for routine immunisations, weighing and developmental checks and can phone the centre for advice. This service is free of charge and care is provided by Maternal & Child Health Nurses (M&CHNs) who are midwives with an additional public health qualification in child development.

her own motherhood experiences with those of her sister and mother, as illustrative of changing social discourses of maternity. A brief literature review is then presented, which draws on a diverse body of literature including writings from the disciplines of medicine, social sciences and psychology. An overview of the study's theoretical framework follows. Chapter 3 presents the study methodology and involves a content analysis of women's stories of motherhood. The sample, data collection and data analysis are then described. Finally, the study's value and credibility are addressed. Chapters 4-7 present the study findings in sequential steps across the study span, from pregnancy to approximately 6-8 months postpartum. Chapter 4 presents 'the project' as the mothering approach favoured frequently by primigravidae over 35, particularly professional women. Chapter 5 presents the transition to motherhood over two junctures. Firstly, maternal experiences over the traumatic first weeks (1-4) are explored. The second juncture (1-4 months) is then presented with accompanying themes of ambivalence and struggle. Chapter 6 presents the 'light at the end of the tunnel' and represents mothering experiences at 4-6 months postpartum. Mothers describe 'giving in' and 'letting go' in a bid to make their lives easier. Chapter 7 represents the final stage of transition to motherhood for the study participants and mothers at this point (more than 6 months postpartum), are overwhelmingly positive about their experiences. They retrospectively report clear stages of maternal identity development. Chapter 8 presents concluding remarks, feedback from the participants and implications for practice, and also proposes areas of further research. The overall importance of the study is then considered.

Summary

In conclusion, this introduction has discussed changing childbearing trends in the developed world, particularly increasing birth rates for mothers over 35 years. This review intended to locate the global nature and extent of changing birth demographics. Although social shifts have given rise to these changes, new trends of later childbearing in the context of maternal employment are, as we shall see later, frequently problematic for contemporary women.

To date, the social context of mothers' lives and socio-political antecedents of mothering have received scant attention. The current study intended to address this breach. In so doing, it was hoped to contribute to the scant body of literature addressing the experiences of contemporary primiparae over 35 and to add to the intellectual debate surrounding the social construction of older first mothering. Finally, it was anticipated that the knowledge gained in this study might have a clinical impact for health professionals and inform strategies for midwives and maternal and child health nurses, in particular, to better meet the care needs of this growing group of mothers.

In the following chapter, a review of the social context of mothering for contemporary women has been undertaken. This review demonstrates that changing social context impacts significantly on mothering experiences.

CHAPTER 2

THE SOCIAL CONTEXT OF MOTHERING

"the meaning of childbirth is interlocked with a society's attitudes towards women" (Oakley, 1979, p. 9)

"[Studies of] ... mothering must take into account the complex relationship of mothering and the material, social ... and ideological conditions in which mothering is done"   (DiQuinzio, 1999, p. 33)

In the 1980s, when I first became a mother, mothering was largely considered to be the next step in a woman's life, following marriage. Choice related to when, rather than if, one would have children. Some 30 years earlier, in the 1950s, the question of when one would have children was never raised. Women simply had children when they married. It was the socially accepted norm. For my mother, marrying in the 1950s, it was expected that she would be pregnant within a year or so of marriage. To be otherwise would raise social questions of aberrant behaviour, faulty physiology or wanton trickery of her husband. Some 50 years later, in 2003, my sister Elizabeth had her first baby at 39 years and, similar to contemporary trends, it was after much discussion, repeated postponement and finally a decision that 'having a baby' was something both she and her husband desired. For each of us mothering represented an entirely different dynamic.

My mother insists that the requirements of her mothering role dictated that we as children should be well fed, clean and respectful to our elders. There was little notion of quality time or infant stimulation, though children were well regarded as innocent and novel. By the 1980s, the social climate was changing, and as a young woman, I was expected to have considerably fewer than my mother's ten children. Later, as a mother, it was my social duty to expend some personal and intellectual effort in raising my children. The notion of fewer, precious children replaced my own experience of being one of hordes of children in the local neighbourhood. Childbearing, however, was considered a normal event and family life with children the correct social pattern. For Elizabeth, having her first birth in the 2000s, maternity was of considerable importance and her infant assumed immense significance as Elizabeth's 'last chance' at maternal experience. In addition to ensuring her infant's health, Elizabeth felt obliged to 'master the task of mothering' and to produce the best baby possible. She also keenly believed in a 'window of opportunity' in which to cognitively stimulate her infant and perhaps augment the child's developing intellect.

Despite contemporary ideas of mothering as a natural, instinctive and 'common sense' role, considerable evidence suggests that mothering is in fact an unstable and dynamic category responding to social, economic and political shifts across time. As such, it is era specific. Just as my mother has difficulty understanding why Elizabeth makes such 'a fuss' about having a baby, Elizabeth, too, believes that our mother, despite raising ten children, has limited understanding of how to raise a child 'properly'. Along with many of her peers, Elizabeth believes that quality time and infant stimulation are really important aspects of child raising. My own experiences as a mother of the 1980s, are located somewhere midway but, for each of us, the requirements of appropriate mothering mean something quite different.

This chapter is presented in three sections. Firstly, the social context of contemporary women's lives and mothering experiences is discussed. Particular emphasis is accorded to the growing selfhood[10] of modern women and conflicting / competing discourses of womanhood / motherhood. Secondly, the literature surrounding mothering over 35 is reviewed and, finally, the study's theoretical framework is presented.

The social context of mothering

In this first section, mothering as a social and dynamic category is explored, followed by a review of the social context of women's lives contemporarily. The growing selfhood of modern women is then presented together with an overview of feminist influence as informing women's individuality. A discussion of competing woman / mother discourses[11], as likely to create tension for mothers, follows. Finally, changing child-raising philosophies and requirements are briefly evaluated as incongruent with discourses of womanhood in an advanced industrial economy.

Mothering as a social and dynamic category

In a process of privileging certain behaviours above others, mothering takes on different meanings historically, which in turn affects the social positioning of mothers (Kaplan, 1992; Smart, 1996). These differing social understandings become apparent when mothering requirements from various historical eras are contrasted. For example, if we compare maternity from late 18th century to the present day, we see 'the mother' transformed from virtual nonentity two hundred years ago to her current position as an all important influence on every aspect of her child's development. This social construction of motherhood is largely invisible, with each era of mothers 'knowing' or seeing the maternal

---

[10] selfhood, in this context refers to a move towards female individuality and life-time possibilities
[11] Discourses, in this context, refers to 'broad social, cultural and historical systems of meaning' Hardin (2001, p. 14).

requirements of their era as the 'right way' to raise children. Every new generation of mothers then assumes the capacity to critique prior generations as 'old fashioned' or as lacking in the modern knowledge that underpins mothering requirements.

This view of dynamic and unstable mothering is not commonly endorsed in the literature surrounding motherhood, most of which suffuses mothering with a mystical quality and presents maternity as something a woman will understand when she becomes a mother. However, within post-structuralist and feminist critiques, the social construction of mothering receives some attention and is largely considered to be dependent on prevailing social discourses. For example, Smart (1996) in her feminist deconstruction of the term 'motherhood', found that changing maternal responsibility related primarily to social change, and Thurer (1994), in her feminist critique of the 'myths' surrounding motherhood, related changing maternal requirements to cultural and social antecedents. Similarly, Dally (1982) and Marshall (1991) considered mothering to be socially constructed and related to parallel social change. Dally also gave mention to changing 'fashions of childcare' historically. Meanwhile, feminists Ehrenreich and English (1988) critiqued the changing 'expert (male) advice' informing maternal approaches during the previous 150 years. They suggested that trends such as scientific and psychoanalytic movements significantly affected mothering discourses.

Currently, Australian motherhood discourses dictate that a mother should be fully committed to the welfare of her infant. Maternal love and devotion are prescribed requirements and child-raising philosophies lean towards a system of intensive mothering, which is further described in a later stage of this chapter. In brief, intensive mothering embodies the notion that children are innocent and precious and require quality interaction and nurturing, preferably by their mothers and most especially during infancy. This, it is believed, is what children need and deserve (Hays, 1996). However, when we contrast contemporary mothering requirements with, for example, attitudes common among 18th century aristocratic French mothers, it becomes immediately clear that mothering requirements are temporally informed. For instance, two hundred years ago motherhood did not exist in any legal capacity and a mother's prime responsibility was the provision of legitimate heirs for her husband (Smart, 1996). It was generally believed that no special attributes were required to raise a child. Good mothering, as we now understand it, characterised by maternal love and devotion, was unknown (Shorter, 1976, p. 168). Abandonment of children was common (deMause, 1974; Fildes, 1990; Hardyment, 1983; Shorter, 1976; Walzer, 1976), as was use of wet nurses (Badinter, 1981; Fildes, 1990; Golden, 1996; Shorter, 1976). Neither practice resulted in overt condemnation of the mother, although high rates of infant mortality were associated therein. Instead of the maternal devotion

21

axiomatic to contemporary mothering, maternal ambivalence was common (Badinter, 1981; deMause, 1974; Pollock, 1983; Shorter, 1976) and Badinter suggests that this ambivalence likely related to views of mothering as a burdensome and dull occupation (pp. 70-71). When we compare these contrasting views of mothering it becomes immediately apparent that 'mothering' as a category is influenced by something other than 'nature' or biology. This indefinable something is the social context of women's lives, which is examined in the following section.

The social context of contemporary women's lives

In order to understand modern motherhood, it is important to look at the social context of contemporary women's lives and there are many factors that contribute to making mothering a very different social experience today than perhaps even 50 years ago. Some of those factors include: mothering in the context of career; the selfhood of contemporary women; mothering as a social choice; competing social discourses of mother versus woman and finally, increasing social importance of the individual child. Each of these factors is considered in the following sections of this chapter.

Mothering in the context of career / work and mothering

In the 1950s/1960s most young women worked briefly, as a stopgap between completion of education and marriage. For my mother, a schoolteacher, marriage spelt the end of her working life. A 'marriage ban' on teaching employment in Ireland in the 1950s meant that female teachers, once married, vacated their position to become a wife and subsequently a mother. Motherhood was central to a woman's life and there was an implicit assumption that all women were or would be mothers, sooner or later. Leaving a paid position for marriage posed no dilemma for my mother or her peers and, among social discourses of the 1950s/1960s, marriage attracted more social status than 'having to work for a living'. Sheridan, Baird, Borrett and Ryan (2002) and Ferguson (1983), who critiqued British and Australian women's magazines of the 1950s and 1960s, found similarly, that marriage and motherhood were essential to the lives of women in this era.

In the 1980s, when I was a young mother, I was working in a part-time capacity as a midwife and I felt confident in my capacity to mother and work outside the home. Unlike my mother but similar to most women of my era, I believed that marriage and motherhood were insufficient destiny for women. My peers and I spoke of making something of our lives and we chose to delay our first births for a couple of years after marriage and to space our subsequent children, which enabled us to return to work between babies. This economic shift towards female employment and mothering in the context of work, particularly part-time work, is abundantly addressed in the literature, for example, Apter (1993); Daniels and Weingarten (1982); Grieve (1986); Kuchner and Porchino (1988) and Wilk (1986). For my generation, although our decisions to work were fuelled in part by a financial need for two incomes, similar to that described within the literature (Filene, 1998; Granrose & Kaplan, 1996; Hattery, 2001; Kuchner & Porchino, 1988), our working choices were also driven by a desire to participate in the public world. While we may not have articulated such a notion exactly, this idea of women working for self-fulfilment first makes its way into social discourses around this time (Filene, 1998). The possibility of 'having it all', that is, interesting and challenging work, sexual happiness, marriage and motherhood (Hoffnung, 1995) also emerged in the 1980s. For myself in the 1980s, there was no question about whether I would work or if I would mother, I would do both. Similar to many of my post-second wave feminist generation, my friends and I understood this to be both our right and our privilege.

By the 2000s, further social changes were evident. For Elizabeth, an industrial chemist, an elective decision to postpone mothering while completing higher education and pursuing career plans marked most of her twelve years of marriage and this trend has become increasingly common among women of the advanced industrial world (Berkowitz et al., 1993; Berryman et al., 1999; Cunningham & Leveno, 1995; Hewlett, 2002b: Hewlett, 2002c; Ozer, 1995). Currently, the vast majority of women work and most well-educated women plan to mother in the context of work / career commitment (Apter, 1993; Benn, 1998; Brown et al., 1994; Hattery, 2001; Hays, 1996). For most women, there is no conflict of interest in postponing first childbearing until their late thirties and indeed, this juncture often represents the first opportunity for pause in a woman's working life, particularly for women who are actively investing in a career. Career structures are, in general, very unforgiving of childbearing / child-raising time out (Hewlett, 2002c).

The most striking difference between the social context of our lives, my mother in the 1950s, myself in the 1980s and my sister in the 2000s, is the social balance we each felt was acceptable, in terms of our mothering / working lives. For my mother, her role as wife and mother was of greater social significance than her teaching work and she uncomplainingly retired prior to marriage. For me, in the 1980s, I considered that work and family were of equal social importance in my life and I accommodated mothering and work, while planning and spacing my children so that it was possible to continue to work. For Elizabeth in the 2000s, the balance was initially weighted in favour of work and career and, although she freely admitted to wanting a baby one day, there was a sense that, while mothering could wait, career opportunities would not. Generally speaking, it is impossible to understand mothering for first-time mothers over 35 without first understanding both the selfhood of

23

contemporary women and the place that work occupies in their lives. This next section aims to explore the question of women's 'selfhood' and work.

The selfhood of contemporary women, work and the feminist movement

No discussion of 'selfhood' for contemporary women could be complete without mention of the second wave feminist movement of the 1960s/1970s, which was perhaps the single most profound influence on 'woman discourses' in first world countries, in the last century. Propaganda of the 1950s, according to Eisenstein (1984), decreed that "femininity lay in clinging to the role of wife and mother" (p. 69), though my mother would describe it differently. This propaganda came under critical review as the social mood swung towards a commitment to female education and equal rights for women, particularly in terms of employment opportunities. Well-educated middle-class women formed the core of this new feminist movement, known for its commitment to female autonomy, both psychological and physiological and also for its commitment to intellectualism. Female solidarity and 'sisterhood' were key themes and, although not all women espoused the 'bra burning' radicalism of this movement, it catapulted the 'women's question' into the public arena and changed forever the way women viewed themselves (Filene, 1998; Gornick, 1996). Women started to think about their individuality and their lifetime possibilities (Filene, 1998; Hattery, 2001) and, for the first-time, the trajectory of a woman's life did not automatically involve only a husband and children. Concordant changes include a more liberal attitude to sexual activity, which was accompanied by the introduction of the contraceptive pill in the 1960s (Filene, 1998; Miller, 1991; Yankelovich, 1974). Twin notions of sexual activity for non-procreative purposes and postponement of pregnancy to fit in with life plans slowly rose to prominence during this era.

Of course, for my mother in Ireland, the contraceptive pill was regarded as the 'devil's own instrument' and its introduction in 'heathen' places such as Britain, the U.S.A. and Australia was greeted in Ireland by Sunday Mass quotations from the Vatican, outlining the 'sacredness of transmission of life' and the sinfulness of thwarting God's plan. Nonetheless, this widespread move towards female equality affected dominant views of a 'woman's place' in society, even in Ireland, and the notion of combining paid work, wifedom and maternity grew along with the consumer movement. There were, expectedly, some restrictions on the sort of employment possible for 'nice' middle-class girls and, of my class of 24 co-students graduating from secondary school in 1977, four employment categories outranked all others: nursing; teaching; the civil service and banking. Indeed, by the late 1970s, the work ethic for young married women in westernised nations, particularly middle-class and well-educated women,

24

changed from 'you may' to 'you should'. Johnson and Johnson (1980) describe a widespread cultural mandate originating at this time, which suggested that intelligent young women should not confine their talents to domesticity and childcare alone (p. 143).

By the mid 1980s, when Elizabeth graduated, further social change was evident and Elizabeth's classmates embraced studies as diverse as law, science and linguistics, in addition to the more usual nursing and teaching. Newspaper and magazine articles of this era feature 'super moms' and 'executive moms' calmly and easily doing it all (Thurer, 1994) and according to Coward (1997) "motherhood [was] is made to look so easy, as if there's [was] nothing involved, no work, no money and certainly no ambivalent feelings" (p. 117). Although Coward's feminist critique does not exactly echo my experiences as a working mother in the 1980s, I am aware of a certain naivety associated with mothering discourses of this era. Images of corporate motherhood, with baby perched on mother's knee between executive meetings, were commonplace and feminist orientated magazines such as Cleo and Cosmopolitan suggested that women could 'do anything'. Other features, in this post second wave feminist era, voiced a concern with social devaluation of traditional stay-at-home mothering roles (Kaplan, 1992).

By the 2000s, subtle yet profound social changes were continuing and the importance of work in a woman's life grew with her job opportunities. For Elizabeth, coming of age in the 1980s and establishing her career in the 1990s, maternity meant something very different than for either our mother or myself. Mothering, for Elizabeth, was viewed as an adjunct to her life, an important adjunct and one at which she was hoping to excel but, nonetheless, an adjunct to her real or important work life. Although this view of mothering as a peripheral addition to a woman's life is not publicly endorsed, it is invisibly inscribed in competing discourses of woman versus mother and the tensions embodied therein are implicated in the maternity / work experiences of contemporary women, most especially women who delay their first births in pursuit of career opportunities. What follows is a review of those competing woman / mother discourses.

Competing discourses of womanhood

In the 2000s, for women like my sister Elizabeth, who had postponed their first births while establishing careers, mothering experiences were often fraught with mixed social messages and competing discourses. A certain degree of tension is evident between discourses of womanhood compared to discourses of motherhood and that tension seems to be largely invisible to women until they too become mothers. These discourses variously suggest that mothering is an important, fulfilling

25

and satisfying experience, that mothering is a socially responsible activity; that mothering is easy and natural but that the infant requires almost exclusive maternal care in infancy in order to grow up well adjusted. Additionally, these discourses suggest that women will live to regret selfish non-mothering choice.

Conversely, womanhood discourses suggest: that women should work; that work is important for women, in terms of self-definition and self-realisation; that a woman's individuality, competition and success in the public world contribute in a socially meaningful way and that maternity alone is considered to be a lesser choice. Tensions related to these conflicting discourses often result in a tendency among women to attempt to 'do everything' and this tendency is most marked among contemporary working mothers. The ensuing 'double burden' has been extensively critiqued by feminist authors, for example, Apter (1993), Eyer (1996), Granrose and Kaplan (1996), Hattery (2001), Hochschild (1989) and Hoffnung (1995).

The origin of this dichotomy can be traced, in part, to second-wave feminism and particularly to the view of maternity as the principal obstacle in the path of women's true liberation (Ehrenreich & English, 1988). Indeed feminism has long had an ambivalent relationship with motherhood (Burkett, 2000; Dally, 1982; DiQuinzio, 1999; Ferguson, 1989). Burkett, who critiqued social discourses around childlessness in American society, eloquently described the relationship as "fraught with resentment over the social prescription that childbearing is women's natural vocation, yet tinged with a keen awareness of the potential power that prescription confers" (p. 150). Other than condemning maternity as the root of women's inequality, the feminist movement of the 1960s/70s showed little interest in the plight of mothers (Coward, 1997) and a tension exists between traditional motherhood and feminism which, to this day, has never been clearly reconciled. In my reading of feminist literature of this era, I find that the question of motherhood is often avoided or insubstantially addressed, and seems to present as something of a 'too hard' question. This tendency towards avoidance also presents in critiques of feminism. Dally, for example, suggests that feminists responded to the mother question by "ignoring and trivializing motherhood" (1982, p. 179), as a way of denying the conflicts mothering posed for women. DiQuinzio (1999) concurred with this finding. Kaplan (1992) actually goes one step further and, in addition to her understanding of an uneasy co-existence between feminism and motherhood, considers that the second-wave feminist movement contributed to the "destabilizing of the mother" (p. 182), by undervaluing mothering alone as a social role.

Although it is not immediately clear that the feminist movement sacrificed the mother in favour of the woman, it is abundantly clear that pre-existing mothering concepts were challenged during this era and

26

a certain degree of female hostility towards domesticity and the institution of motherhood subsequently emerged. From this time, mothering alone, although still a socially important role, occupied a lesser role for women than did success in the public sphere. Social shifts such as increasing consumerism and an expanding industrial economy also gave rise to increasing female employment and a lessening of social expectations around 'stay-at-home' mothering (Apter, 1993; Sheridan et al., 2002; Summerfield, 1998). In addition to trends of decreasing family size and delayed first parturition, notions of childbearing as a social choice emerge around this time.

Childbearing as a social choice / to mother or not to mother

"Childbearing has become a matter of choice rather than destiny, deliberation rather than duty. One in five women, we are constantly told, will not even have a child. She has got other things to do."

(Benn, 1998, p. 29)

Within the literature, the notion of childbearing as a social choice first made its way into mothering discourses of the 1980s (Daniels & Weingarten, 1982; Kuchner & Porchino, 1988; Wilk, 1986), most likely related to a growing sense of female individuality. Although present from this time, the notion of non-childbearing choice within marriage or stable partnered situations, was not well regarded in public discourse and associations of selfishness, high-income status and high level of career achievement were common (Marshall, 1993). Mothering in the 1980s, I was not aware of the possibility of choosing not to have children. It simply never entered my mind, though my sister, coming of age some five years later, understood delaying childbearing in pursuit of career opportunities to be a reasonable choice. Later in the 1990s, Elizabeth describes discussing with her husband whether or not to have children, but the discussion occurred only after repeated postponement of childbearing. This trend of repeated postponement, succeeded by a decision not to have children is noted in the literature (Hewlett, 2002c; Kuchner & Porchino, 1988) and Hewlett has coined the term a "creeping non-choice" in recognition of this tendency (Hewlett, 2002b, p. 9).

Whatever the origin, it is clear that an element of choice entered mother discourses in the 1980s and this choice included the question of whether or not to mother, or indeed in what social context to mother. A concomitant change of mood, towards a time when childbirth and childcare were no longer automatically regarded as an integral part of a woman's life, is noted in the literature (Dally, 1982; Kaplan, 1992; Kuchner & Porchino, 1988). Strangely enough, at the same time as this shift towards female employment, career opportunity and childbearing choice was occurring, a parallel and confusing move towards 'natural childbirth' and 'intensive' mothering is noted. The paradox arises from the expansion of the mothering role at a period when considerably less maternal time is available.

27

Notions of natural bonding and female self-reliance also prevailed from this time and are discussed in the following section, as contributing to the dilemmas many modern mothers face.

Natural childbirth

Thurer provides a good, if cynical, summary of the 'natural birth' movement of this era:

"Women who had babies in the 1970s wallowed in the aesthetics of it all, natural childbirth and nursing were maternal musts. The institutionalisation of baby slings to keep baby close, the obsession with mother-bonding, 'rooming-in' in obstetric units, the video-taping of the birth experience for posterity, all attest to the ... infatuation with the concept of tender-hearted, empathetic child rearing." (1994, p. 260)

This movement promoted birth as 'natural' or 'instinctual' and most probably arose in response to a growing disenchantment with the medicalisation of childbirth. Oakley (1984), for example, lent the movement some momentum with the publication of her book "The Captured Womb" in which she critiques patriarchal obstetric interventions (p. 249). Martin (1987), too, is scathing of traditional notions of the uterus as "involuntary muscle" doing the work of labour, and argued instead that the woman was more than a passive observer in the process (p. 58). Women of this era (late 1970s/1980s) were now increasingly portrayed as in tune with and reliant on their bodies' natural propensity to birth. There was a sense of reclaiming birth for women as a natural and 'powerful' womanly achievement and, as a midwife during this era, I became intimately familiar with 'new' birthing options such as birthing stools, bathtubs and beanbags on the floor. Women were encouraged to mobilise during labour and to adopt a position of comfort for birth, instead of the more common supine bed bound position. The usual enema and shave fell into disrepute and by the mid 1980s were outlawed except for operative delivery.

Notions of maternity as a source of womanly fulfilment, achievable no other way, emerged in the 1980s as an extension of the natural birth movement. Successive authors, such as Barlow and Cairns (1997), Marshall (1991) and Kaplan (1992) make note of this changing social mood and move towards a view of maternity as a source of satisfaction for women. An attenuation of radical feminism over the preceding decade may also have made space for this changing view. From my own reading of post-second wave feminist literature, mothering took on a different social value at this stage and was now deemed "not bad, just insufficiently valued" as Coward (1997, p. 116) declares. This understanding represents a change of mood from earlier feminist understandings of maternity as an impediment to womanly self-actualisation. Marshall (1991), in her review of mothering manuals of the 1980s, provides a useful summary of this mood:

"The experience of childbirth, having a newborn baby and the process of childcare are all described in exalted terms. It is emphasized that this is a special experience, being essentially creative and positive…the end result is ultimate fulfilment for women which can be gained no other way."   (p. 68)

Other changes traceable to this era and enormously affecting mothering expectations for subsequent generations of birthing women, was a resurgence of interest in natural mothering as accompanying natural birth and a new interest in the father as a parent (Thurer, 1994). The birth of a baby came to be viewed as a shared parental experience (Stoppard, 1983; Thurer, 1994) and it was now politically correct to have father present in the birthing room, helping his partner through the trials of labour and symbolically cutting the cord thereafter. A resurgence of interest in breastfeeding is also traceable to this era and campaigns such as 'breast is best' were used to promote public awareness of the benefits of maternal nursing. Breastfeeding became endorsed as an integral part of good mothering, but also took on a mystical quality, as enabling the mother to 'do the right thing'. The following quote from La Leche League is something of an exemplar:

"Mothering includes not only feeding the baby, but keeping him warm and comfortable, soothing his feelings of fear and anger… the deepest, truest spirit of mothering grows as you experience the quick, strong feeling of affection so natural between a nursing mother and her baby … this sensitivity which helps you to do the right thing at the right time, which comes from knowing him, develops from spending time with him and it develops more quickly and to a certain degree, if you are nursing your baby." La Leche League (1977, pp. 9-10)

As will be clear from the women of this study, this notion of breastfeeding as the 'right way' to feed a baby places enormous pressure on contemporary older first-time mothers, many of whom struggle to lactate. This difficulty is further addressed in chapter 5.

Along with the growth of the natural birth movement, a change in childrearing philosophy becomes evident from this time. This new child-raising philosophy was both labour intensive and costly and was likely driven by trends of fewer precious children and a rise in the social importance of the individual child. A requisite increase in maternal time and effort accompanies this model of child raising and impacts significantly on the workloads of contemporary women who strive to do justice to both work and child raising.

Intensive mothering: the provision of 'quality time'

" … the qualitative importance of socialization during the early years of the child's life has acquired a much greater significance than in the past – while the quantitative amount of the mother's life spent either in gestation or child rearing has greatly diminished"

(Mitchell, 1971, p. 172)

The social importance of the individual child has risen in accordance with declining family sizes and currently a model of intensive mothering is widely endorsed in advanced industrial nations. This model involves a parenting style that is active and striving and is largely considered to be laughable by my mother and her peers, mothering in the 1950s. For them, the requirements of mothering were that children should be clean and well cared for, and the notion of children having 'needs' was scarcely entertained. Quality time or infant stimulation received scant attention and my mother declares that we, as children, turned out all right without all that 'parenting'. Although I can acknowledge that we did indeed 'turn out alright', as a mother of the 1980s, I have to admit that I feel this relates as much to good luck as to good guidance and, in common with my own peers, I strove to provide some 'quality' time for my children, during their early years. Attendance at swimming classes, pre-school learning centres and the provision of reading and activities at home were included among my efforts. For Elizabeth, mothering in the 2000s, her mothering experiences acquired an intensity above and beyond that experienced by myself or our mother and Elizabeth was keen to cognitively stimulate her infant in a bid to avail of a postulated receptive time in her infant's development. This my mother interprets as a terrible fuss and, although I understand Elizabeth's impetus, I too consider that she is needlessly creating work for herself.

In general, this trend towards ever more intensive mothering seems to be driven socially by several factors, including principally: concerns around the safety of children; advancement of the consumer movement; and greater competition for scarce educational opportunities and career pathways. It becomes important that children have the best possible opportunity for advancement and this notion is accompanied by an understanding that children are innocent and in need of protection. Hays provided a particularly useful summary of this child-raising model:

"The model of intensive mothering tells us that children are innocent and priceless, that their rearing should be carried out primarily by individual mothers and that it should be centered on the child's needs, with methods that are informed by experts, labor intensive and costly. This, we are told, is the best because it is what children need and deserve."

(Hays, 1996, p. 20)

Within this model, there is an assumption that the child requires constant and consistent nurturing, particularly in infancy, and the mother is considered to be the person best fitted for this role (Forna, 1998; Glenn, 1994; Hays, 1996). An accompanying component of cognitive development, unheard of in previous generations, has been adopted and mothers of the 1980s/1990s were expected to stimulate and develop their children to their full potential. In an extension of this notion, Thurer (1994) describes the use of flash cards and cassettes, in the U.S.A., aimed at giving children a head start. This model of mothering is often embraced by well-educated women, and it follows that older professional mothers, who have considerable disposable income and who aspire to models of excellence, are likely to subscribe to this model of child raising.

Both socially and within the realm of my midwifery practice, I am particularly struck at the intensity mothering seems to invoke among contemporary mothers, especially professional women. A friend provides a useful case in point. Julie[*] is 37 years old and a fulltime computer specialist, and she struggles to do justice to the various requirements of her life. To accommodate 'quality time' with her infant son, she has condensed her work into 4 days, though in reality this means working until midnight at least 2 days a week. On her Wednesdays off, Julie devotes the day to her son Harrison and in fact refers to Wednesdays as 'Harrison's time'. On those days she turns off her phone, refuses to switch on her computer and takes Harrison to a giddy range of activities, including gym sessions, swim classes and mothers' group. On Thursdays, Julie returns to work, secure in the knowledge that she is 'doing the right thing' by her son.

Understandably, for women like Julie, tensions between her views of being a 'good mother' at the same time as being a 'good worker' create anxiety as she tries to accommodate 'everything'. This increase in maternal anxiety, related to women's struggles to not only 'do everything' but to also 'get it right', is found within the feminist literature addressing contemporary mothering, for example, Hattery (2001), Hays (1996), Rubenstein (1998) and Thurer (1994). This incongruence between women's social expectations of fulfilment through participation in the public sphere and the intense requirements of the mothering role is central to the research question raised in this study and is addressed throughout this work. First, however, it is important to appraise the literature pertaining to mothering over 35, particularly as it informs and guides health professionals involved in the care of this group of mothers.

Transition to motherhood literature

In this section, the transition to motherhood literature is reviewed as a means of establishing current knowledge surrounding first mothering over 35 years. It is important to state that this overview of the literature is not exhaustive and that more detailed review has been attended throughout the findings chapters. The aim of this brief review is to present some of the categories of literature addressing mothering, particularly older first-time mothering, and to then outline particular deficiencies in the body of knowledge. To date, much of the research literature relating to pregnancy in women aged over 35 years focuses on the associated medical risks of delayed childbearing. One might indeed ask why

---

[*] pseudonym

this is important or of what relevance medical research is, in a study concerned with the social context of mothering for contemporary women. However, we will see in later chapters that this perception of risk does indeed impact significantly on maternal experience for this group of women. For that reason, a brief summary of the medical research literature around older mothering is now attended.

Medical research

Overall, medical research into older childbearing seems to support an established link between advanced maternal age and a panoply of increased risks which include: high blood pressure (Barton et al., 1997; Kullmer, Zygmunt, Munstedt & Lang, 2000), pre-eclampsia (Barton et al., 1997; Sibai et al., 1997; Tan & Tan, 1994), gestational diabetes (Bobrowski & Bottoms, 1995; Dildy et al., 1996), chromosomal abnormalities (Dildy et al., 1996; Hollier, Leveno, Kelly, McIntire & Cunningham, 2000; Luthy, 1999) and low birth-weight infants (Aldous & Edmonson, 1993; Bonellie, 2001; Cnattingius et al., 1992). Additional risks for this group include unexplained fetal death (Anderson et al., 2000; Cnattingius et al., 1992; Fretts, 2001), uterine dysfunction during labour (Main, Main & Moore, 2000), pre-term delivery (Cnattingius et al., 1992; Lehmann & Chism, 1987; Roberts, Algert & March, 1994; Tan & Tan, 1994) and increased risk of operative delivery (Kullmer et al., 2000; Main et al., 2000). Nevertheless, although undeniably associated with increased risk of fetal compromise, the actual statistics relating to fetal morbidity for the older mother do not significantly differ from those of her younger counterpart.

This theme of greater risk without actual increase in infant morbidity figures is repeated in several studies. Prysak, Lorenz and Kisly (1995), found that although nulliparae[12] over 35 years had higher rates of pre-natal, intra-partum and neonatal complications than average aged nulliparae, there was no increase in perinatal mortality rate. Spellacy, Miller and Winegar, (1986), in a study of 511 mothers over 40 years, found that although older women of normal weight and low parity showed higher rates of diabetes and caesarean delivery than their younger counterparts, their infant outcomes did not differ significantly from the younger women in the control groups. Smit, Scherjon and Treffers, (1997) found that, after selection for low risk, elderly nulliparae did not have an increased incidence of fetal distress or other emergency factors compared to the younger control group. Pollock (1996) found "no clearly demonstratable adverse outcomes" to be linked to the infants of primiparae over 30 years (n = 4315) in a U.K. study (p. 429). Meanwhile, Roberts et al. (1994) concluded that women who give birth after 35 years of age faced increased risks but that these risks were largely manageable in light of modern care.

---

[12] women who have not yet delivered a child

Similarly, Dildy et al. (1996) found that pregnancy in the 45-50 year age group was generally safe in the absence of pre-existing medical disorders. Overall, there is a general understanding of older maternity as hazardous but manageable with advanced obstetric care. What is not clear from the literature is to what extent risk relates to pre-existing maternal compromise, such as chronic hypertension and diabetes or to lifestyle influences, such as smoking, maternal weight and general health. Research into the real risks of maternity in a healthy older cohort is one area requiring further attention.

Now, in the following section, studies of mothering are evaluated as it is important to establish the extent of the body of knowledge surrounding mothering, particularly first-mothering for women over 35.

Studies of Mothering

Existing studies of mothering tend to fall into two broad categories. The first of those categories includes studies that view motherhood from the perspective of maternal infant attachment (Gottlieb, 1978; Tulman, 1981) and are underwritten by understandings of attachment / separation (Ainsworth, Yarrow & Glaser, 1962; Bowlby, 1953) and maternal infant bonding (Klaus & Kennel, 1976). The second category covers those studies that examine maternal role attainment and, because the interest of this study is firmly located in mothering experiences and maternal role attainment, this category is of greater interest. Studies, such as those conducted by Rubin (1967a, 1967b, 1984) and Mercer (1986) were particularly influential in the field of maternal role attainment and are thus reviewed here. Rubin explored the cognitive and social processes involved in maternal adjustment and discussed a process of claiming the infant as fundamental to maternal role attainment. Meanwhile Mercer (1981, 1985, 1986) understood maternal role attainment as an incremental, developmental process, with the mother becoming attached to her infant over time as she gained confidence in her mothering role. Theories of transition are also commonly utilised to explain maternal role achievement (Cudmore, 1997; Leonard, 1993; Pridham & Chang, 1992; Rossi, 1968; Sethi, 1995) and are under girded by understandings of sociological work from the 1950s and 1960s.

Nursing research presents another area of mothering literature and authors such as: Barclay, Everitt, Rogan, Schmied and Wyllie, (1997); Ferketich and Mercer (1990); McVeigh (1997a, 1997b); Pridham and Chang (1992); Reece (1995); Tarkka and Paunonen (1996) and Tarkka, (2003) often present a more practical angle on mothering adjustment and the stresses therein. These studies frequently discuss factors that assist or hinder maternal adjustment, such as maternal and infant characteristics, social and family support for the mother and prenatal hospitalisation or stress. A significant body of nursing research examines maternal adjustment and the experiences of mothers with ill or pre-term infants (Doering, Moser, & Dracup 2000; Hurst, 2001).

However, according to Rogan et al. (1997), nursing studies of mothering rarely "move beyond description" and, additionally, seldom address maternal transition (p. 879). Rogan et al, further found that nursing research in this area was heavily influenced by "medical and psychological" approaches to mothering (p. 879). Indeed, in the past twenty years, the psychological experience of mothering has received some attention and authors such as Barlow and Cairns (1997), Leifer (1980) and Stark (1997) explored the meaning of motherhood, particularly first motherhood for women. Much of the mothering literature, however, examines maternal adjustment among average-aged mothers and does not feature age-related comparisons.

Mothering over 35 years

Literature searches revealed a dearth of qualitative research into older first-time mothering. Studies located included: a small number of doctoral studies, undertaken in American universities (Dobrzykowski, 1998; Nelson, 2003a; Smith-Pierce, 1994; Twiss, 1989) in the disciplines of sociology, psychology and nursing; one study addressing stress and older primiparity (Reece, 1995) and a study addressing changing demographics associated with later first-time mothering (Ventura, 1989). Other studies focusing on mothering over 35 years include a small body of comparative studies, examining maternal adjustment among younger and older mothers, for example, Gottesman (1992) and Mercer (1986) and a number of studies relating to older mothers, though not confined to first-time mothering (Berryman, 1991; Berryman et al., 1999; Berryman & Windridge, 1995, 1996; Dobrzykowski & Stern, 2003; Ragozin, Basham, Crnic, & Robinson, 1982). Despite a link between older primiparity and higher than usual levels of anxiety (Steinberg & Bellavance, 1999; Stowe & Nemeroff, 1995; Windridge & Berryman, 1999) and prominent suggestions of higher levels of maladjustment and postnatal depression, when reviewing the literature, it became clear that little was known about the actual experiences of motherhood for primiparae over 35 years. Specifically, the socio-political and cultural antecedents of maternal adjustment are not well addressed and few studies have concentrated on the social context of contemporary mothering, particularly for first-time mothers over 35.

The challenge for this study was to locate a framework that was sufficiently broad ranging to address the complexities of first mothering for women over 35 years and to also permit an exploration of the social context in which new mothering occurs. Specifically, the resulting framework sought to address

34

an understanding of the individual as being influenced by the various expectations / requirements of his/her life as opposed to common humanistic views of the self as autonomous and self-determining. For those reasons, a post-structural approach was employed which was additionally informed by the tenets of feminist theory, as sympathetic to the lives of women.

Theoretical framework

The theoretical approach of this work hinges on an understanding of the 'performance of self' that is located within post-structural thought. The individual is presented as being shaped by the discourses in which he/she participates, rather than as a unitary subject. Congruent with the discussion of changing women's life trajectories and social antecedents above, social discourses are now presented as central to the construction of the post-structural self. In this context, discourses refer to "broad social, cultural and historical systems of meaning, creating both the notion of 'self' and how the 'self' constructs its world", as described by Hardin (2001, p. 14). The 'self' within post-structuralism is then explored, together with subjectivity[13] as a mediating factor in this view of 'self'. Finally, a brief overview of feminist theory as it contributes to the theoretical framework for this study is presented.

Discourses in post-structuralist inquiry

"The political and other arrangements typical of a society are implicated in the conventions of discourse."

(Rosenwald & Ochberg, 1992, p. 265)

Discourses can be understood as interconnected systems of social meaning (Lupton 1998) which can be traced historically, thus locating how particular sets of knowledge and behaviours have evolved (Gastaldo & Holmes, 1999). Indeed, Gastaldo & Holmes suggest that discourse "can only be understood in the context of historical development of a given society" (1999, p. 232)and it is through the interaction of power and discipline within a society that certain discourses are privileged and rise to eminence. Thus, particular social trends emerge. In this sense, social discourses are reflective of power equations within societies (Gastaldo & Holmes, 1999; Gubrium & Holdstein, 2000) and, as vehicles of power, discourses are constitutive of the individual in a fundamental way. The political arena from which they arise also affects emergent or changing discourses. For example, an interest in saving mothers arose in the years immediately following World War 1 in England, in recognition of the importance of mothers for the future of the race (Lewis, 1980). There is little doubt that this elevation

---

[13] Danaher, Schirato, and Webb, describes subjectivity thus "Subjectivity is the term derived from psychoanalytic theory to describe and explain identity, or the self. It replaces the commonsense notion that our identity is the product of our conscious, self governing self, and instead, presents the individual identity as the product of discourses, ideologies and institutional practices." (2000. pp. xiv-xv).

35

of maternal importance and changing maternal discourses related to a sense of urgency to replace lives lost in the war and a political preoccupation with under-population.

From a post-structuralist view, a discourse is always spoken about in reference to a discursive object. For example, discourses of motherhood are structured around the child, society and appropriate maternal behaviour. Each discourse has a particular viewpoint on how to define and understand behaviours (Hardin, 2001). For instance, changing discourses of the last century have elevated the importance of maternal love and devotion, to a point where it is now believed that maternal dedication and nurturing are imperative for the child's normal development. In possession of this knowledge, individual women shape their behaviours to commonly understood meanings of motherhood. Although social discourses do not exist merely as social guides to appropriate behaviour, it is through these discourses that individuals come to know what is expected of them socially and how they should behave in particular circumstances, such as mothering.

One of the key issues in transition to motherhood is the accommodation of the maternal self and the incorporation of this strand into the woman's previously held personal sense of self. Indeed, issues of self are so clearly central to the women's stories in this study and so clearly related to prevailing discourses, that it is opportune at this juncture to examine the nature of self that is particular to post-structuralism, in the context of this research.

The nature of self that is particular to post-structuralism

As a key concept within post-structuralism, the 'self' assumes a particular importance as being formed through the discourses of the day. This formation occurs within social and cultural boundaries, a notion endorsed by post-structural authors. For example, Davies suggests that "one can only ever be what the various discourses make possible and one's being shifts with the various discourses through which one is spoken into existence" (1991, p. 43). Butler (1990) too, supports this view, suggesting, "… the 'doer' is invariably constructed in and through the deed" (1990, p. 142). Within post-structuralist thought, twin notions of power and discipline are omnipresent and Foucault's writings, in particular, present a case in point. Foucault suggests that social discourses "systematically form the objects of which they speak" (Foucault, 1989/1972, p. 49) and understands that relationship to be one of disciplinary power:

" … it is … one of the prime effects of power that certain bodies, certain gestures, certain desires, come to be identified and constituted as individuals. The individual, that is, is not the vis a vis of power; it is, I believe one of its prime effects. The individual is an effect of power and at the same time, or precisely to the extent to which it is that effect, it is the element of its articulation"

(Foucault, 1980, p. 98)

At this stage it is also useful to mention Foucault's understanding of governmentality as a vital concept in fashioning the self. For Foucault, governmentality was comprised of two distinct strands. The first strand relates to politics of the state and "bio-power", or more simply population management, in terms of the governing of individuals and the creation of "docile bodies" (Gastaldo, 1997, p. 114). Within this view, normative standards of behaviour are produced socially, through the power of disciplines such as medical and educational institutions and through a series of 'technologies' of classifying, disciplining, and normalising (Danaher et al., 2000; Mansfield, 2000). For Foucault this complex power was invested in institutions and processes:

"... the ensemble formed by the institutions, procedures, analyses and reflections, the calculations and tactics that allow the exercise of this specific albeit complex form, which has as its target population, as its principal form of knowledge political economy" (Foucault, 1991, pp. 102-103)

The second strand of governmentality, which is of considerably more interest to this study, is the micro level of what Danaher et al. consider 'body politics' (2000, p. 83) or the conduct of the self. The relationship we have with our own selves and also the relationships in which we participate with other individuals shape every aspect of our lives. As Foucault explains:

"We are the inheritors of a social morality which seeks the rules of acceptable behavior in relations with others"

(Foucault, 1988b, p. 22)

Categories of difference and comparison such as mad/sane, sick/well, criminal/non criminal present within Foucault's work and, according to Foucault, these categorisations urge individuals to work on themselves, and thus comply with standards of normality within their culture.

Fittingness of approach

This idea of being constituted through discourse is peculiar to post-structuralist thought and is in stark contrast to commonly held humanist views of 'self' endorsed by westernised cultures. The humanist view subscribes to the belief that individuals make free and autonomous decisions in their lives, possessing, as Hardin suggests, "the capacity to ascribe private meanings to life circumstances and [to] make choices based on those meanings" (2001, p. 13). Although many women in advanced career structures would indeed consider that they make free and autonomous decisions in their work and lives, this view may actually be counter-productive within their mothering experiences, in denying the powerful social influences underpinning motherhood. If a woman believes that she can plan and control her mothering experiences, then she may not address the limitations of her 'choices' and may also feel personally responsible for each minor difficulty she encounters. Although it is not the intent of this work to present the self within post-structuralism as in binary opposition to the humanist self, it is useful to consider the contrasting conceptualisation of mothering post-structuralism offers. This conceptualisation is chosen here as a fitting way to explore the social tensions underlying the experience of mothering for contemporary women over 35 years, particularly women used to agency and autonomy in the public sphere.

The self as a performance / subjectivity

In post-structuralist tradition the 'self' is actively constructed and temporally contingent. Within this view, the self is not so much an entity as an activity or, as Hardin suggests, "not a thing but a performance" (2001, p. 14). Thus, the self is actively fashioned through discursive performance, with largely invisible discourses influencing the 'choices' individuals make. Foucault explains:

" The political and social processes by which the Western European societies were put in order are not very apparent, have been forgotten, or have become habitual. They are part of our most familiar landscape and we don't perceive them anymore."

(Foucault, 1988c/1982, p. 10)

Additionally, because individuals are discursively formed as both self-aware and self-reflective (Davies & Harre, 2001), they possess the ability to see themselves objectively or from outside, described by Hardin as "someone else's subjective 'taking in' or 'gaze'" (p. 13). More simply, this refers to seeing oneself from someone else's point of view. A second aspect is that of taking the objective, or that outside of oneself, "internalising it and making it subjective" and thus incorporating it into one's self (Hardin, 2001, p. 13), meaning that humans behave as they expect others to view them. This is perhaps the key concept of post-structural subjectivity. By virtue of being both subject and object, individuals possess the ability to gaze at themselves and to monitor their own behaviour. A key aspect of performing the self involves this tailoring of oneself to normative standards. Self-monitoring occurs silently and unknowingly and individuals censor their actions against contemporary normalising standards of behaviour "as an exercise of self upon self" (Foucault, 1988a/1984, p. 2). Social rewards for adhering to 'normal' codes of behaviour influence individual action (Hardin, 2001) and we are all familiar with the exclamation of 'what would people think!' as individuals position themselves within boundaries of 'normality' and make sense of new life events. A prime motivation for adhering to normative codes of behaviour is, according to Hardin, to "avoid the consequences of being labelled abnormal" (2001, p. 16). Thus, categories of difference such as good and bad, inscribed in cultural understandings, inform the individual's behaviours. In this study, categories of difference related

38

principally to social discourses of good/bad mothering, and women struggled to adapt to prescriptive maternal behaviours associated with good mothering.

In the following section, feminist theory, as sympathetic to the challenges of women's lives, and as addressing the complexities of interviewing women around an emotionally charged subject, such as childbearing, is discussed as it informs this study's theoretical framework.

Feminist Theory

"... feminist thought is necessarily concerned with the relationship between social positioning, experience, knowledge, interests and action"   (New, 1998, p. 351).

Although feminist theory emerged largely in response to perceived patriarchal philosophies that rendered women invisible (Jaggar & Young, 2000), it has led to a valuing of women's experiences and an understanding that women view the world differently than men (Ezzy, 2002; Finch, 1999; Reinharz, 1992). It is this understanding that the current study invokes. Additionally, feminist research is generally concerned with the everyday lives and experiences of women (Kvale, 1996), which is in keeping with the intent of this study of women's experiences of mothering. Finally, the feminist understanding of an existing relationship between social positioning and experience, described above by New (1998), is an important component of this study's framework.

Feminism and post-structural theory, points of convergence

In this work, both post-structural theory and feminist theory are drawn upon and inform the study's theoretical framework. This merger is a common one within feminist literature (Butler 1992; Riley 1988; Scott 1992) and focuses primarily on the use of language in the construction of femininity (Scott 1996; Wagner 1995). Originating in France, circa 1970s, and influenced by theorists such as Foucault, Lacan, Derrida, Irigaray and Kristeva, post-structuralist feminism offered an opportunity to critique totalising forms of feminisms (Friedman 1995; Wagner 1995). However, the intent of this study is not to problematize feminism's varied forms or roots, but to invoke St. Pierre & Pillow's (2000) understanding of post-structural and feminist theories as two theories that "work similiarly and differently to trouble foundational ontologies, methodologies and epistemiologies" (p. 2).

Although briefly considered in an earlier section of this chapter, feminist literature is reviewed here for its significant contribution to the way in which many modern women view mothering. Authors such as De Beauvoir (1952), Friedan (1963) and Greer (1970) were dismissive of patriarchal notions of a 'woman's place' in society and the meaning of maternity in a woman's life. In particular, the notion of mothering = womanhood, which pre-existed the 2nd wave feminist movement, came under critical review during the 1960s/1970s. Oakley (1974; 1979; 1981; 1984; 1986; 1992) has been especially influential in this regard and is well known for describing adjustment to first mothering as almost universally problematic (1979, 1986), a previously little voiced notion. Rich (1977) also made a major contribution to mothering literature and was perhaps one of the first writers to discuss the 'institution of motherhood' and to explore mothering from the perspective of the mother. The cultural expectations of the mothering role is another area receiving some attention (Benn, 1998; Crouch & Manderson, 1993; Hays 1996; Thurer 1994) and, although this area is not exclusively addressed by feminist literature, it tends to lean towards that orientation and is thus grouped here. The social 'myth' of mothering, which views women as innately maternal and willingly sacrificial is also critiqued by feminist authors, for example, Forna (1998), Glenn (1994), Hays (1996) and Thurer (1994).

In sum, the key characteristic of this framework is the post-structuralist approach, wherein the individual is viewed as being shaped by the discourses of the day. Within largely invisible social discourses, self-monitoring occurs and the self is fashioned to cultural standards of normality. In this way, the self is considered as a performance rather than a fixed entity. Finally, feminist theory contributes as understanding of the lives of women and as appropriate for researching sensitive topics such as childbirth.

Summary

In conclusion, this chapter has discussed mothering as a social and dynamic category, influenced by cultural, social and political antecedents. A review of the social context of women's lives contemporarily has argued that changing life trajectories for women considerably influence maternal expectations and subsequent experience. The developing selfhood of women, related to increased participation in the workforce and higher education, and influenced by tenets of second wave feminism, was also acknowledged. Competing woman / mother discourses were then reviewed, as likely to create tension for modern mothers. Mothering discourses of the past few decades have not, in general, kept pace with changing social roles for women, and the implications for conflict between the public and private roles of women have never been greater. Current child-raising philosophies endorse a system of intensive active mothering as the best way to raise a child, but this trend is curiously at odds with women's changing social roles. Present-day mothering requires selflessness from women who have been socialised as individuals through their school and work experiences. The difficulties are further heightened by the fact that, although much lip service is given to the importance of mother-work, work in the public sphere attracts more social prestige.

How society views mothers and mothering has enormous implications for women of today, who may be considering whether or not to have children. The social expectations of the role and the possibility of reconciling it with women's private aspirations are factors affecting decisions around childbearing and women's subsequent transition to motherhood experiences. Thurer (1994) describes the dilemma exactly in the following quote "motherhood versus personal ambitions represents the heart of the feminine dilemma" (p. 287). Further, a review of the literature relating to mothering over 35 years reveals a dearth of qualitative research. In particular, the social context of mothering is poorly attended. In the final portion of this chapter, the theoretical framework of the study has been presented, informed by understandings of the post-structural self as fashioned through the discourses in which the individual participates. The feminist component of this framework has also been elaborated, particularly as it relates to a valuing of women's accounts. Finally, it is important to state that the function of this research is not to portray the mother over 35 as a mindless follower of fashion, but to suggest that a tension exists between conflicting expectations of mothering / womanhood in advanced post-industrial nations.

In the following chapter, methodological and conceptual issues are discussed. In particular, Hardin's (2001) methodology is explored, as informing the current study. This particular approach recognises that all individual accounts are located within a matrix of interconnecting social discourses.

CHAPTER 3
METHODOLOGY

" The main interest in life and work is to become something you were not in the beginning. If you knew when you began a book what you would say at the end, do you think you would have the courage to write it?"

(Foucault, 1988c/1982 pp. 9-15)

In the course of this study, the methodological approach has undergone major revision many times and, indeed, seems to have taken on a momentum of its own in response to unanticipated events encountered along the way. Like Foucault's statement above, the direction it has taken has been both transformative and unpredictable, and the resulting methodological approach presented here has evolved in response to the challenges of the study. This research sought to explore the manner in which motherhood was taking place in Melbourne, Australia, in 2002/2003, for a new social category of women, first-time mothers over 35 years. The women of this study, like Elizabeth in chapter 2, had mostly postponed childbearing whilst completing higher education or pursuing career opportunities, and this trend is increasingly common in advanced industrial nations. As we shall see in this chapter, the study sample and later discussion of participant characteristics are reflective of contemporary parturition trends.

It has been argued in the previous chapter that changing maternal life trajectories impact significantly on women's experiences of motherhood. It has also been demonstrated through the stories of three women of my family, that cultural and social antecedents powerfully shape women's understandings of appropriate mothering. In a bid to critique broader social, historical and cultural discourses underlying maternal experience, a post-structural approach has been used in this study. In particular, the methodology outlined by Hardin (2001) as "embracing individual stories yet recognising that all stories are nested within a background of broader social and cultural discourses" (p. 11) is drawn upon. This methodology takes a particular view of the self, not as a unified and static being but as a dynamic being, who is shaped and reshaped by the discourses in which he/she participates. In addition, storytelling and the sharing of stories are commonly considered to play an important part in the way individuals make sense of life experiences (Bruner, 1986; Davies, 1991; Gergen, 2001; Holstein & Gubrium, 2000) and, for that reason, the utility of stories in shaping the social self and the mother is reviewed here.

In this chapter, there are seven main areas of attention. Firstly, storytelling as a means of interpreting life events is reviewed, together with the methodology employed by the current study. Secondly, the sample is presented in terms of size, recruitment criteria and recruitment strategies. Thirdly, data collection through interviewing is presented. Fourthly, the researcher's own struggle to position herself within the research is addressed followed by a discussion of ethical concerns. Sixthly, data analysis is described, followed by a discussion of issues of value and credibility for the current study. Finally, the participants are presented in self-described groups as a preliminary to the ensuing findings chapters.

Storytelling and self construction

"Self narratives function much like morality tales within a society ... they are cultural resources that serve such social purpose as self-identification, self justification, self-criticism and social solidification." (Gergen, 2001, p. 249)

Language is a central concept in the construction of the post-structural self and is reflective of historical, cultural and social context (Bruner, 1984). As such it contributes to common understandings of behaviour (Hardin, 2001). As a primary means of communication, the language and exchanges in which people engage, both between and within themselves, are always dependent upon available discourses, and thus, resultant stories reflect common cultural and temporal understandings. Individuals are constructed socially through the stories they tell and the self is shaped, refined, reinforced and adapted to prevailing cultural norms. Rehearsing and telling the story of 'self' facilitates reflection and the development of new ideas. This notion of the contemporary self as being constructed through storytelling is well supported within sociological, feminist and socio-linguistic literature, as is the belief that storytelling occurs within cultural and social boundaries (Bruner, 1984; Chase, 1995; Davies, 1991; Davies & Harre, 2001; Gergen, 2001; Holstein & Gubrium, 2000; Rosenwald & Ochberg, 1992; White, 1981). Although the available social discourses may not differ within a cohort, stories are constructed differently, depending on which discourse the teller invokes, and resultant stories are tailored to the lives of the participants (Chase, 1995; Davies & Harre, 2001). Holstein and Gubrium describe this notion exactly, suggesting that "narrators artfully pick and choose from what is experientially available to articulate their lives and experiences" (2000, p. 103). Individual stories are broadly similar while at the same time differing in their particulars.

In addition to understanding that one can only ever be what the various discourses allow, within post-structuralism there is room for changing or even conflicting accounts to be articulated, as individual viewpoints shift and alternate discourses are invoked. The availability of alternate discourses is not unlimited, however, and peer pressure is one way in which availability is affected. Holstein and Gubrium (2000) show a particular understanding of this notion, suggesting that "self construction orients broadly to the interpretive mandates, controls and constraints of group membership" (p. 105).

For example, it is expected that contemporary Australian mothers should be fully committed to their infants and put their infants' needs before their own. This social belief forms a particular curb, in dictating 'appropriate' maternal behaviour to women.

An important point to make at this juncture is that individual stories do not exist in isolation, but as Bruner suggests "must be seen as rooted in society and performed by individuals in cultural settings" (1984, p. 5). In this way, stories connect individuals to their culture and cultural practices, and as Sandelowski suggests, "provide a sense of connection to other people"(1994, p. 26). This connection occurs in daily transactions and the self is rehearsed and tailored to prevailing discourses. Ordinary stories and exchanges in everyday life are of particular importance in enabling individuals to make sense of the world. Indeed, Bruner (1986) discusses the especial importance of everyday "epiphanies" in this context (p. 13). Another interesting aspect of the stories people tell, is the temporal location of those stories, described by Bruner as "historically positioned in a given time, place and social moment" (1984, p. 5). In the following section, the function of stories as a 'snapshot' in time is discussed.

Stories as a snapshot in time

"A life story or self story is still a story, a representation of a life at a given moment rather than the life itself"

(Sandelowski, 1991, p. 163)

Within post-structuralism, stories are understood as providing temporally significant meaning and as being related to cultural norms (Bruner, 1984; Carolan, in press-a; Hardin, 2001). Thus, stories provide a snapshot in time. For this study, participants' stories are presented as a picture of first-time mothering for women over 35 in Melbourne, 2002/2003. In this context, articulated stories are understood as created fictions, which are reflective of the participants' current experiences. Accordingly, the stories do not present a single unified 'truth' which is in keeping with post-structuralist tradition. However, despite being 'mere' verisimilitudes, life-stories are not diminished in importance and Bruner argued that the knowledge derived from stories, though quite different from more highly valued scientific knowledge, performed an equally essential role in facilitating self-understanding (1986, pp. 12-13). Summerfield (1998) enlarged on this view, suggesting that personal stories were actually the product of the "relationship between discourse and subjectivity" (p. 16), a notion endorsed by the current study. Here, stories were sought as a valuable means of accessing the social context of the participants' lives and the meaning of mothering in their life trajectories. The intended focus is congruent with Hardin's suggestion that the analytic focus should not be so much on which story is 'true', but on how stories perform truth (2001, p. 12).

44

Finally, it is commonly held that storytellers select the elements of the stories they tell in order to present their 'slant' on events, a notion commonly found in the literature (Bailey & Tilley, 2002; Goffman, 1969; Summerfield, 1998). For some, this might suggest that the use of stories as data is problematic. However, despite the notion of a personal view within stories, there is a co-existent understanding of common social and theoretical underpinnings among even the most diverse stories (Hardin, 2001). To quote Holstein and Gubrium "... as they actively craft and inventively construct their narratives, they also draw from what is culturally available, storying their lives in recognisable ways" (2000, p. 103). It is this very point of common underpinnings that makes the use of stories a worthy choice for the current study. Although stories of transition to motherhood are likely to and indeed do vary, there are underlying commonalities. There is an emphasis on performing motherhood, within available discourses, as participants struggle to position themselves within their new role. This study's methodology draws on stories as a means of making sense of life events and the evolving method is described in the following section.

Evolving method, study rationale

The original intent of this study was to conduct in-depth interviews and analyse those interviews using content analysis. However, as we shall see in a later section of this chapter, earlier plans to remain objective at interview proved difficult and a move towards reciprocal and interactive interviewing resulted. This evolving interview format gave rise to conversational data, which were more like stories than 'objective' data, and I began to consider the meaning of stories in women's lives. Sandelowski's work, in particular, was inspirational and the evolving method was informed largely by a reading of Sandelowski's many publications and earlier understandings of thematic and content analysis. The eventual method, content analysis of the women's stories, was considered a useful and meaningful way of examining the social context of participants' mothering experiences and is similar to methodologies employing content analysis described elsewhere, for example, Downe-Wamboldt (1992) and Bowling (2002).

Furthermore, normalising discourses produce certain 'truths' in our everyday lives, which are nonetheless difficult to access, as largely invisible and 'taken for granted' beliefs, which are often uncritically accepted as 'common sense' (Crowe, 1998, p. 339). Some of these beliefs have, to use Forna's wonderfully expressive idiom, been so long unchallenged as to be "woven into the fabrics of our consciousness" (1998, p. 2).

As this work unfolds we will see that in using this post-structuralist methodology, connections between personal accounts and broader cultural and political discourses could be sought. Thus, identification of the interpretive framework used by individual mothers to make sense of events in their lives became possible and underlying social discourses could be exposed for critique. The rationale for this methodology is encapsulated within Ezzy's belief that, in order to understand the meaning of something, the researcher must "locate the event ... in a broader narrative that defines its purpose and therefore its significance" (2002, p. 95). Finally, this methodology considers the positioning of the researcher within participant interviews, a salient point for studies informed by feminist theory. Therefore, a qualitative method, employing in-depth interviews and informed by the researcher's feminist views is an especially suitable methodology, fitting well within the post-structuralist intent of the research. In the following segment, the participants are presented in terms of sample size, selection criteria and recruitment. Data collection methods are outlined and the researcher's rationale for recruitment and sample size are made explicit.

Sample

According to Sandelowski (1995b), a common misunderstanding in qualitative research is that sample size is not very important (p. 179) and, although a variety of guides exist to assist the beginning qualitative researcher, it is difficult to gauge appropriate participant numbers. Additionally, qualitative studies vary considerably in sample size, from as few as four participants to as many as forty. For the current study, an extensive review of the literature revealed a plethora of suggestions as to what constituted appropriate sample size. Rice and Ezzy's suggestion that "a sample size is sufficiently large when the researcher is satisfied that the data are rich enough and cover enough of the dimensions they are interested in" (1999, p. 46), was used as a guide to sample size. It was anticipated that a purposive sample of 18 women who met the selection criteria would be recruited. The number 18 was chosen as representative of many similar qualitative studies.

Recruitment and rationale

A purposive sample of older first-time expectant mothers [aged over 35yrs] was recruited through the admissions office of the tertiary level hospital where the researcher works. Approximately 3,500 pregnant women attend this hospital annually for care and women from a wide range of social backgrounds and ethnicities are represented. For this study, participants were recruited on the basis of age primarily and it was expected that a range of socio-demographics would be represented in the sample. However, although access to all women delivering at the hospital was permitted, when I came to recruit participants I found that the majority of primigravidae over 35 years attending the hospital had private insurance and attended a private obstetrician for care. These women planned to deliver in the private unit attached to and sharing facilities with the tertiary hospital. Of women aged over 35 years, delivering in the public hospital, most were having a fourth or fifth baby rather than a first and, despite efforts, few women satisfying the inclusion criteria were found in the public sector[14]. In the final sample, one participant was cared for as a public patient.

Additionally, it was anticipated that there would be some participants who were single mothers and some who were in same-sex relationships, in line with growing trends of differing family configurations in advanced industrial nations, such as Australia. The eventual sample, however, consisted predominantly of middle-class white women in heterosexual relationships. One woman from a same-sex relationship provided a single exception. There were no single mothers in the sample. Participants included 2 Australian born Chinese women, a single Australian-born Indian woman and one participant from Sri Lanka who had come to Australia 4 years previously. During the recruitment period there were no black women attending the hospital for care who satisfied the selection criteria and although there were 4 overseas born Asian women who otherwise met inclusion criteria, none spoke sufficient English to be included in the study.

As discussed in chapter 1, this trend of older first-time mothers as more likely to be well-educated and financially secure (Berryman et al., 1999; Berkowitz et al., 1993; Ventura, 1989) was also my experience of recruitment. In Australia, subscription to private health insurance is positively related to increasing age [over 23 years] and higher income level (ABS, 1995). Employed women over 35 years are thus considered likely to have private hospital cover. As discussed earlier, well-educated women are also associated with greater use of healthcare systems (Morrison et al., 1989; Najman et al., 1998; Raum et al., 2001). It is therefore likely that a private hospital, sharing facilities with a tertiary level public hospital, caters well for this particular segment of the population.

Participants were recruited in the following manner. Pregnant women attending maternity booking interviews at the hospital are routinely given information folders regarding visiting hours and information such as necessary clothing and equipment for baby. During recruitment for this study, an

---

[14] In Australia, all citizens are entitled to free medical care in the public hospital system. This system operates on a clinic basis and patients are seen by available and mostly junior doctors, who are overseen by a more senior specialist. Hospital admission is on a similar basis and hospital stays in public hospitals are generally considerably shorter than in private hospitals. Many middle class individuals choose to pay for private health insurance, which allows them to see a private doctor of their choice and attend a private facility for care and thus avoid lengthy waits in clinics.

47

information leaflet outlining study details, was included in the information folder for each woman who met the inclusion criteria, described below. These information leaflets outlined the study, likely time requirements, details of the voluntary nature of participation and also a contact number to express interest and seek more information. Inclusion criteria included:

- First-time mothers
- Aged 35 years or older at time of booking
- Uncomplicated pregnancy
- No major underlying medical complication
- English speaking

As the primary interest of this study was the transition to motherhood for this cohort, women with serious underlying medical conditions, such as cardiac disorders, were excluded, as were women whose babies were expected to have significant disorders, as it was likely that such serious conditions may have coloured the perception of birth and adjustment in these women. Similarly, non-English speaking women were not recruited due to the expected difficulty of accessing their accounts. It was anticipated that there would be some difficulty recruiting sufficient numbers for the study, which was both lengthy and time consuming. However, this was not the case. Participants already recruited sought other participants from among friends and acquaintances. Women delivering in other hospitals, who had heard of the study through friends, phoned to express an interest. Several women delivering a second baby, but who otherwise satisfied the criteria for inclusion approached to offer their stories. A final sample of 22 women aged over 35 resulted, over-recruited to cover expected drop-outs. The expected loss of participants, however, did not occur and only one participant was lost to the study, due to a move overseas.

As the study progressed and themes emerged I became increasingly concerned that the emerging categories did not relate entirely to age, but also to career structure, so with permission from the university and the hospital, an additional sample of five primiparae aged approximately 30 years, to represent average age of childbearing in Australia (ABS, 2000), was recruited purposively. These women were chosen on the basis of significant investment in education / career, as below. Women satisfying the criteria were approached on admission to hospital and their participation invited. The original information leaflet was given to these women. Women interested in participating contacted the researcher and a time for interview was arranged, as with the older group. Criteria were as above with the following exceptions:

- Aged approximately 30 years

- Significant investment in career development, defined as tertiary professional qualification or degree and employment in the chosen field.

Data collection

Interview 1	Interview 2	Interview 3
35-37 weeks gestation	10-14 days postpartum	6-8 months postpartum
30 minute contact interview	1 hour in-depth interview	1 hour in-depth interview
Themes for discussion	Themes for discussion	Themes for discussion
Demographic information	Birth experience	Motherhood experiences
Preparation for mothering	Early mothering	What information, if any, might have helped?

In this longitudinal study, an initial contact interview was conducted at approximately 35-37 weeks gestation and was timed to hopefully coincide with the participants' commencement of maternity leave[15]. At this interview, demographic information such as educational standard, work / career status and duration of current relationship was gathered and hopes and expectations for the forthcoming birth were discussed. Two in-depth interviews followed. The first in-depth interview was conducted at around 10-14 days postpartum, to capture the birth experience and experiences of early mothering. The final interview was timed to occur when the infant was approximately 6-8 months old. This timing was chosen to coincide with a less stressful juncture, when the infant was hopefully sleeping through at least occasional nights, as suggested in the literature (Kerr, Jowett & Smith, 1996; Wolke, Sohne, Reigel, Ohrt & Osterlund, 1998). It was further anticipated that, by this time, participants may have had an opportunity for reflection on their experiences of motherhood.

---

[15] In Australia, maternity leave is generally unpaid and women may legally take one year of leave and return to the position they previously held. It is recommended that expectant mothers take a minimum of 6 weeks prior to the anticipated birth and the remainder after the infant is born.

In a bid to create as natural and familiar an environment as possible and to facilitate the woman's convenience in caring for her infant, interviews were conducted in the women's homes. Audiotaping of the interviews occurred with the participant's permission. Prior to interview, a theme list was mailed to each participant [Appendix A]. Although initially the interview schedule was planned to include three interviews, when I actually started to interview the women I found the initial interview largely superfluous and the elicited information was almost universally repeated at the second interview. I had felt it was important to be known to the women prior to delivery and not simply arrive unannounced at a vulnerable stage in the new mother's life. However, the women did not share my reluctance, but were eager to talk and 'debrief' about their experience. Therefore, after a total of 5 pre-natal and 5 postnatal interviews, a decision was made to dispense with the initial contact interview and thereafter participants were interviewed only twice postpartum, as per schedule.

Interview format, rationale and methodological strengths

In-depth interviewing was chosen as a pertinent vehicle of inquiry in line with Kvale's (1996) understanding of in-depth interviews as "conversation that has a structure and a purpose" (p. 6). This type of interview focuses on the participant's perception of self, his/her life and experience, expressed in his/her own words. The particular interview format here was informed by Patton (1990) and influenced by Ellis, Kiesinger and Tillmann-Healy (1997). This approach permitted:

- a list of questions/themes to be explored during interview
- spontaneous generation of questions in pursuit of interesting material that emerged unexpectedly
- data gathered to be different for each interviewee;
- interviewer responsiveness to situational changes;

(Patton 1990, pp. 281-287).

The approach has also been influenced by Ellis et al. (1997), who espoused a feminist orientation and suggested interactive interviewing as appropriate for researching "emotionally charged and sensitive topics" (p. 121) such as childbirth. Some characteristics of interactive interviewing include:

- a joint effort by interviewers and interviewees to understand the phenomenon
- sharing and telling of stories and developing a relationship similar to the way in which relationships develop in real life
- the researcher's own feelings are explored and add validity to the study
- researcher's self disclosure is encouraged

50

- interactive and non-hierarchical/dialogic rather than interrogation
- views similarities such as cultural ethnic and gender between the interviewer and interviewee as important
- may provide a therapeutic benefit to participants

(Ellis et al. 1997, pp. 121-124).

In this study, interviews evolved into an informal conversational format, with a particular interest in creating a collaborative exchange of ideas. This type of interviewing allowed the participants' views to unfold in their own words and permitted a valuing of women's accounts, which is in keeping with feminist tradition. Non-hierarchical interviews employed here were also in keeping with feminist theory (Oakley, 1981). Fontana and Frey (1998) understood this notion well and found that by moving away from hierarchical interview schedules, women were more likely to digress into their personal lives and histories. For the current study, this particular method was also considered likely to be acceptable to women aged over 35 years, many of whom had previously held positions of seniority in the working world. It was anticipated that an egalitarian and collaborative approach might be congruent with the women's life and work experiences. Another important consideration was that this format permitted probing, which greatly assisted access to the meanings participants ascribed to their experiences. This, according to Marshall and Rossman (1999), is central to good qualitative research. Interviews were also flexible and sensitive to the dynamics of each interaction and were tailored to specific encounters, which allowed pursuit of interesting information that arose unexpectedly. At the same time, this approach acknowledged the sensitive and emotional nature of childbearing.

This particular method of interviewing is also useful when participants are to be interviewed more than once. Friendly conversational type interviews allow a relationship to develop between the researcher and participants, similar to the way in which relationships develop between friends (Ellis et al., 1997). In general, rapport building is considered important in securing the long-term interest of participants (Ellis et al., 1997; Oakley, 1981). In this study, it was hoped that, in collaborating and exchanging ideas, participants would feel part of the research, rather than simply being the 'researched'. Finally, the longitudinal nature of this study was considered advantageous in that it facilitated correction of earlier omissions and offered a second opportunity to pursue information. Later interviews thus provided an opportunity to build on participants' earlier interviews, to seek clarification or to plot changing views. For this study, positioning of the researcher was also considered to be an important part of the developing method and is discussed as follows.

Positioning of the researcher in the research

As a beginning researcher, I agonised over my early interviews with new mothers and found it well nigh impossible to pitch interviews to my satisfaction. I was keenly aware of the advice offered by the many research books and interview guides I had consulted. Maintaining a friendly distance was prominently advised. Discussions with other qualitative researchers and attendance at a 'conducting qualitative research' course suggested that one should not be drawn into venturing one's own opinions, but instead the researcher should gently steer the interviewee back to the subject by saying something to the effect of 'what I'm really interested in is your opinion on this matter'. Thus, I entered the interview situation with pre-conceived ideas of how I would conduct the research, mindful of the fact that my voice should not be overly present in interviews. Rather my role was to prompt, probe and stimulate the interviewee's account of her experiences. Later, when I came to transcribe these early interviews I was shocked to discover how audible was my voice. I had slipped effortlessly and unconsciously into my clinical midwifery role. The women repeatedly asked my advice and I responded as a midwife, offering information on breastfeeding, infant settling and other concerns they voiced. How to reconcile my two roles was something that consumed my thoughts and I struggled to find an acceptable compromise. Finally, after a great deal of thought, reading and discussion, I came up with reciprocity as the key to making the interviews work and simply responded to the women as a researcher, a midwife, a woman and a mother, in fact, as a human being, with all the attendant complexities.

Reciprocity

Reciprocity ... "means building in ways to promote mutuality, equality and sharing between the researcher and the participants ... [and] involves negotiating all aspects of the relationship ... between researcher and participants."

(Fahy, 1997, p. 33)

Reciprocity was an important component of developing relationships between the participants and myself. As a midwife employed in the care of parturient women, my approach has always been to answer women's questions honestly and empathetically and I found I was unwilling to move from this stance. I was also keenly aware that my status as a midwife, at the hospital where the women gave birth, greatly facilitated my entrée into the interview situation. I felt that providing some advice when requested, or answering questions as they arose, greatly increased the women's receptiveness to my questions. During the course of the interviews I found the women asked many questions and sought reassurance on issues as diverse as sudden infant death syndrome [SIDS] to the optimum time to wean. I answered the questions as they arose and returned to my theme list as soon as practicable, feeling that it would be morally indefensible not to reassure a clearly anxious woman when it was within my capacity to do so. Oakley (1981) found with this view, declaring that, in women's interviews, there could be 'no intimacy without reciprocity' (p. 49) and it was my understanding that interviewees expected a certain amount of reciprocity from me, as a midwife and as a mother. Alvesson and Skoldberg (2000) too, concur with this notion of intimacy and reciprocity and stress the necessity of "establishing a close and mutual relationship between researcher and subject" (p. 215) in order to successfully interact with participants.

Indeed, much of the feminist literature suggests that women respondents are keen to share their experiences with a woman researcher (Finch, 1999; Oakley, 1981; Reinharz, 1992) and particularly so, if she shares some life experience with them (Wasserfall, 1997), as I do, being of a similar age, class and gender as the participants. Additionally, as a mother, the women were particularly receptive to my 'understanding of motherhood'. Thus, when the women asked, I told them something of my own mothering experiences and shared tips that had worked for me and worries I had experienced as a new mother. Often, I volunteered the information without being asked. In my opinion, engaging in empathetic sharing made the interviews more honest and morally sound, a finding supported by Fontana and Frey (1998).

Overall, I was surprised to find that the participants of this study were so keen to speak to me, as the project was both time-consuming and lengthy. Indeed, such was their eagerness that a simple phone-call to arrange an interview appointment often took 30-40 minutes, as the women told me of their experiences to date. Frequently, when I attempted to explain the purpose and necessity of consent forms the women tried to wave them away and said 'I trust you' or something to the effect that the tabloids would not be interested in their mundane experiences. Like Finch (1999), I had expected to spend time establishing a rapport. Instead I was invited into the women's homes and offered tea/coffee. Because many of the interviews occurred at around 11am, I started to bring scones for morning tea. This seemed to set the meeting off on the right foot and allowed us to get acquainted socially before launching in to the interview. As an icebreaker, I usually made small talk before starting the interview and I would endeavour to make my position clear, as a benign and approving presence. In fact, I became 'someone who understands', to use the phrase so often repeated during the interviews. I frequently reiterated how exhausting and difficult new motherhood was and my understanding of insufficient social valuing of this important role. Just as in my clinical practice, I used humour to ease tension as participants were often a little tense initially. Almost always, I admired their babies and commented on how well they looked. Only on one occasion have I been worried about an infant and, with the mother's permission, I called the maternal and child health nurse. The women showed me around their nurseries and displayed the gifts friends had bought for the babies. Often, it felt like I was visiting a friend who had just had a baby. Sometimes, I was asked to hold the baby while the woman made tea, other times I offered to hold a fractious baby and slipped quietly into my midwifery role. Frequently, the women told me it was like talking to a friend and that the time went really quickly. Repeatedly, I sensed their reluctance to end the conversation and many times I was invited to call or phone if I needed any further information. A couple of times I've had to restrain myself from offering babysitting or other assistance, as the short intense relationship we shared felt like a friendship.

Acknowledgement of the women's emotional fragility was important and I felt that a degree of flexibility and sensitivity was required to address these issues. During the interviews I used personal anecdotes and stories, which in my opinion are a valuable tool in allowing vulnerable women to admit to feelings they consider 'unworthy'. I frequently solicited information by commencing a sentence thus 'several of the other women on the study experienced … and I wondered what is your experience of that?' Knowing that 'feelings' of that nature were experienced by others had the effect of giving permission for disclosure. Sometimes, I used humour to talk through the 'perfidy' of human nature and transmit my view that mothering was a difficult and exhausting task for the new mother and also that it was possible to love one's baby and still feel short-changed by expected sacrifices. Sometimes I would talk 'through the baby' to the mother, for instance if the baby was particularly fractious and the mother was becoming agitated as she tried to convey to me how much she was 'in control' of the situation. I would say to the baby, something to the effect of 'oh, give your poor Mum a break' and effectively change the focus from maternal to infant behaviour. I would follow it up by making a comment such as 'nature had made a wise choice in allocating the care of infants primarily to mothers, as the continuity of the race would not otherwise be secure'. Thus the women's accounts became stories, similar to the stories friends exchange and not, as anticipated, question and answer type exchanges. Finally, due to the short intense relationship shared by participants and the researcher, a certain degree of closure was required at study's end.

Closure

At the completion of the study, participants and their, by now, toddlers were invited to an afternoon tea at the hospital with the researcher. An overview of the study's main themes was mailed to each participant approximately two weeks prior, and mothers were given an option of returning the comment sheets by mail or at afternoon tea [see Appendix B] Study findings were discussed on this occasion and an opportunity to ask questions was provided. The afternoon tea was attended by 18 of the 22 mothers, all of whom expressed pleasure at having being included in the study. Several felt that the study had been worthwhile in terms of feeling that their experiences as new mothers were valued and also in allowing them to reframe their experiences of early mothering favourably. Others suggested that the afternoon tea provided an opportunity to network with other participants.

Although the women's stories make up the larger part of the research, focus groups of health professionals were also conducted prior to participant interviews, in a bid to frame the research question more clearly. Focus group recruitment, data analysis and findings are presented in Appendix C.

Ethical considerations

Following university and hospital ethics approval, recruitment of participants was attended as previously described. Issues of consent and participant confidentiality were dealt with as follows. Consent was obtained at first contact from all participants and the option to withdraw from the study at any time for any reason was reiterated during recruitment and prior to each interview. Focus group participants were similarly advised that participation was voluntary and the option to withdraw was offered prior to each group discussion. Participant confidentiality for all participants, mothers and infants, midwives and M&CHNs has been protected in this study through the use of pseudonyms and participants were advised prior to participation that this measure would be in place.

Concerns

One ethical concern that arose during the course of this study was the unanticipated development of a friendship-type relationship between the researcher and participants. Within post-structuralist principles friendship is largely considered a performance, thus, it begs the question- 'how does the performance of friendship affect (a) the data gathered and (b) the analysis of that data?

In the performance of friendship, in this case, a potentially unequal friendship with myself, as researcher and possibly as clinical expert, and participants who may have been intent on projecting a certain image, several possible dilemmas emerged. For example,

1. Was there a risk of recruiting biased data as participants' strove to give appropriate responses?

2. Did this format of relaxed and friendly interviews encourage a level of disclosure that the participant might later regret?

3. Was there a greater risk of participant exploitation, dependent on an engaged and interactive research relationship?

In her account of feminist ethnography, Stacey (1991) considered that the research process, in it's dependence on human relationship, engagement and attachment... places research subjects at grave risk of manipulation and betrayal" (p.113).

After considerable reflection, I came to understand that it was simply not possible to guard completely against the recruitment of potentially 'biased' information in this study. Further, I consider all information to be context based and in this case, I believed the data was shaped by the interview situation, the interviewer, and miscellaneous other influences, such as the current level of fatique the new mother was suffering. Thus, my approach was to consider all information as a snapshot in time, and although subject to the vagaries of that particular moment, likely underpinned by common cultural understandings as described earlier in this chapter (Holstein & Gubrium, 2000).

The notion of presentation of the 'right story' also arises and is further explored in chapter 5. Concerns that the relaxed interview format employed here might result in a level of disclosure that participants might later regret were ameliorated by realising that this level of disclosure seldom leads to participant distress (Weiss 1994, p.123). Indeed, it is commonly considered that the research relationship might offer "helpful support as a respondent explores matters that had been confusing, distressing or painful" (Weiss 1994, p.123), a finding supported by Ellis et al., (1997).

With regard to data analysis, I felt, like Robson (2002), that "knowing what distortions and biases we are likely to introduce in our observation should help us in countering them" (p.322). With this in mind, I strove to understand my own position and my contribution to the interview situation and this notion of researcher transparency is more fully considered in the following section.

Researcher transparency

Reflexivity: "An acknowledgement of the role and influence of the researcher on the research project. The role of the researcher is subject to the same critical analysis and scrutiny as the research itself" (Rice & Ezzy, 1999, p. 257).

Researcher transparency is frequently advised as a check of trustworthiness (Alvesson & Skoldberg, 2000; Hertz, 1997; Sandelowski, 1986; Scott, 1997) and, in this study, two areas are presented for attention. They are: reflexivity and the provision of an audit trail. For the purpose of this discussion, Rice and Ezzy's description of reflexivity, as above, is used. The provision of an audit trail is considered at a later stage of this chapter. What follows now is a discussion of reflexivity, for the context of this research.

Reflexivity

Overall, the idea of researcher impact in qualitative research is not new and Geertz explored the notion as early as the 1960s (Geertz, 1963). In his later work, Geertz is particularly scathing of the suggestion that ethnographic researchers must be objective and scientific (Geertz, 1988). Within nursing research, the concept of reflexivity is relatively recent (Koch & Harrington, 1998) but gaining momentum. Interaction between the researcher and the data is increasingly recognised as important (Cutcliffe, 2000; Ellis et al., 1997; Okely, 1992; Rice & Ezzy, 1999; Turner, 1987). There is, however, no real consensus on the importance of researcher impact, and conflicting views of the value of the researcher's previous knowledge and experience persist. Traditionally, qualitative research has been plagued with such doubts (Morse, 1991). Some methods advocate acknowledgement of personal beliefs and subsequent holding in abeyance of those views (Polit & Hungler, 1993), lest the researcher "perceive a mirror image of [his/her] hopes/fears and not the social reality" (Cutcliffe, 2000, p. 1479). Others, such as Lipson (1991), suggest that reflexivity centres on the researcher being part of the data, rather than distant from it. Researcher objectivity and removal from the qualitative situation is increasingly seen as unlikely and even counter-productive. Chesney (2000) suggests that the researcher's philosophy and beliefs "form the bedrock on which the choice of method is based" (p. 59), while Alvesson and Skoldberg (2000), believe that emotion is inevitable and a vital part of the researcher's interest and motivation.

Although there is no clear consensus within the literature on just how the researcher influences the research situation, it is clear that qualitative research is socially constructed (Mulhall, LeMay & Alexander 1999). Therefore, it follows that the researcher's philosophy and values and the context of the research may affect the chosen methodology and, ultimately, the interpretation of findings. In that context and bearing in mind that any authored work bears the mark of the person who created it (Erlandson et al., 1993), it is important at this juncture to examine my own position within the research (see also Carolan 2003a).

Upon reflection, I am aware that my background as a midwife and mother and my philosophical stance, values and feelings have undeniably contributed to the interest I have developed into the experiences of older first-time mothers and also to the way I view childbearing and motherhood. I acknowledge that my particular stance is pro-natalistic, but I also feel that motherhood is a difficult and onerous

57

responsibility, for which there is insufficient social value or recognition, which in turn contributes to the angst many new mothers, particularly first-time mothers over 35, feel. My personal feminist leanings have also contributed to a valuing of women's experiences and an endorsement of non-hierarchical models of care. Self-understanding is generally regarded as an important pre-requisite to understanding the impact of the researcher on the data and more particularly on the research participants and thus the phenomenon under review. Additionally, within post-positivist research, there is a recognition that all research emanates from a particular ideological viewpoint, which in itself is not problematic, once acknowledged (Scott, 1997). Self-reflection addresses this issue by allowing the researcher to become acquainted with his/her own philosophical stance.

Finally, a general critique of positivism has, according to Alvesson and Skoldberg, (2000), also lent emphasis to the value of the "researcher's whole person" (p. 218). I found this notion of the researcher as a 'whole person' particularly interesting, as the tension I felt initially within the research situation related to role conflict, research / clinical / social roles, rather than encompassing my person as a whole. I came to realise that the angst I felt as a neophyte researcher related to concerns of not 'doing the research job properly' or 'colouring the data with my presence and values'. In pursuing the notion of reflexivity, I learnt that contemporary thought embraces such 'colouring' of data as a 'good thing' and endorses the richness and insight it affords.

In the following section of this chapter data analysis of all data is reported.

Data Analysis

All data from the current study, including interview and focus group transcripts [see Appendix C], were processed in the same manner, involving transcription, reduction of data and data analysis.

Transcription and data reduction

In this study, audiotapes were listened to repeatedly in order to get a sense of the content. Full interview and focus group texts were then read several times, over several weeks. Data reduction commenced when the researcher felt confident that a reasonable understanding of the underlying stories had been achieved. First, interviewer questions and comments were deleted. In removing interviewer comments and questions the data was immediately reduced by approximately one third. Next, words that detracted from the key idea of each group of sentences were also removed. These removed ideas and words were filed together for later review and the remaining text was read and re-read for content. Further reduction took the shape of removal of extraneous participant comments such as 'umm,' 'well now' and 'you see' and the resulting individual stories were shaped for coherence. The above steps were repeated until the stories were reduced as much as possible, without sacrificing content. Individual stories were constantly compared to the full text to check and recheck content. The following step involved content analysis of the shortened stories.

Content analysis

"...content analysis is used to refer to any qualitative ...sensemaking effort that takes a volume of qualitative material and attempts to identify core consistencies and meanings"

(Patton, 2002, p.453)

The analysis in this study was orientated to the informational contents of the data and was interested in identifying core consistencies and meanings, as described by Patton above, Bryman (2001) and Downe-Wamboldt (1992). Qualitative content analysis employs a system of coding and measurement (Morgan, 1993), identifying units of analysis (Downe-Wamboldt, 1992; Graneheim & Lundman, 2003; Krippendorff, 1980), which in this instance, were indexes of feelings, events and thoughts. As such, the analysis conforms clearly to the tenets of qualitative content analysis as described by Cavanagh (1997), Clifford (1997), Downe-Wamboldt (1992), Graneheim & Lundman (2003), Holsti, (1969), Morgan (1993), Patton (2002) and Robson (2002).

Bearing in mind that repeated readings and close attention to data, together with rigorous transcribing, often lead to insights that ultimately shape the presentation of data in text (Ezzy, 2002), I began data analysis early, transcribing audiotapes verbatim and reading the transcripts, usually the same day, but always within days of the interview / focus group. I personally transcribed all the audiotapes, which I felt was important in acquainting myself with the content of the women's stories and data from the focus groups. This attention to transcripts facilitated reflection as did keeping a journal and discussion of emergent themes with subsequent participants.

Although three stages of data management are described here, all steps proceeded concurrently and thoughts of what it all meant filled my head throughout this stage. I encountered my first major hurdle following transcription and data reduction and I experimented with several approaches before settling on one for the next stage. First I made hundreds of notes and memos about the possible meanings of various similar statements. Then using different coloured highlighters to identify themes and fragments of related themes, themes were coloured and moved together to form an amalgamation of related themes within each individual story. Traditionally, qualitative data has been hand sorted and coded in this manner (Bowling, 2002; Clifford, 1997) and according to Bowling, this attention to detail has the

59

advantage of the researcher "maintaining a close relationship and awareness of the original data"(2002, p.345), which was my intent. In order to remain focused, I also constantly asked myself how did these women describe themselves and mothering?

Each woman's story yielded somewhere between 4 and 8 themes and these themes were then separated out of the individual stories and amalgamated with similar themes from other stories. For example, the theme of 'finding my own way' presented time and again in the women's stories as a way of moving forward from the fears and uncertainty of early mothering. Each time I came upon this theme I highlighted it green. Later, I moved all the green highlighted themes together. During this step, my thoughts were influenced by my reading of Rowe's (2003) qualitative study of infant sleep patterns. In that study, Rowe described presenting fragments of stories recruited during in-depth interviews and shaping them into related themes. This is what I did. This process of moving fragments of related themes together was repeated several times in the current study until only interrelated themes and fragments of themes remained.

Several academic colleagues and texts advised 'immersing' oneself in the data, though initially I was unsure of what this meant. Finally, I came across Orona's account of data analysis, where she described allowing the data to "float" about and to be thus absorbed into her awareness (1990, p. 1249) and that is what I did. I spread the related themes, in an array of glorious highlighted colours, together with the original transcripts across the office to get an overview of the entire transition. I took notes and jotted down thoughts. I tried to visualise how the various parts contributed to the whole. By reading and re-reading the themes and keeping track of thoughts and reflections by means of a journal, I traced new emerging sub-themes. In this way, data analysis proceeded through three increasingly higher levels of abstraction similar to that described by Clifford (1997). Throughout, I discussed my ideas with colleagues and my supervisor and, indeed, anyone I knew who had even a passing acquaintance with the world of mothers and babies. In this way, finally, five interweaving themes emerged from the data:

- The project 'doing it properly' / 'getting it right'
- Vulnerability and anxiety
- Finding my own way / challenging expectations
- The importance of work / balancing work and family
- The meaning of being an older mother

However, although these interweaving themes were entirely true to the data, they did not tell the whole story. A stronger message seemed to be the temporal sequence of transition to motherhood and a decision was made to elucidate the findings in sequential phases. Findings are presented in chapters 4-

7, using this format. This approach sits well with the sequential order suggested by maternal life trajectories, discussed in chapter 2.

In the next section of this chapter, issues of study value and credibility are addressed, followed by a presentation of the participants as a prelude to the findings chapters.

Value and credibility

Qualitative research is based upon the belief that there is no one single truth, rather that the social world is multi-faceted. However, like Hammersley (1992) I felt that researchers should make some effort towards establishing credibility, otherwise there was a danger of conjuring up concepts. My efforts towards establishing credibility were influenced by Sandelowski's (1986) understanding of credibility below:

"... a qualitative study is credible when it presents such faithful descriptions or interpretations of a human experience that the people having that experience would immediately recognize it from those descriptions or interpretations as their own. A study is also credible when other people can recognize the experience ... having only read about it in a study"

(Sandelowski, 1986, p. 30)

Within qualitative literature, approaches to credibility present no clear consensus of opinion. Appleton (1995) suggests enlisting the aid of an experienced colleague to verify categorisations and concepts, though Cutliffe and McKenna (1999) consider this approach to have major philosophical flaws, claiming that such a view endorses a belief that if more than one person agrees with a category then this must be more accurate than a single categorisation. Others, such as Speciale and Carpenter (2003) and Koch (1998), suggest leaving an 'audit trail', or pathway of analytic decisions, which can be followed by another researcher. Still others suggest that by making explicit the researcher's position within the research, the credibility of the findings is increased (Altheide & Johnson, 1994; Andrews, Lyne & Riley, 1996). Self-reflection or reflexivity, as a means of understanding the impact of the researcher's views and values, is thus seen as a valid means of adding credibility and value to qualitative research. Indeed, Alvesson and Skoldberg (2000) attest that self-reflection and the critical self analysis of feelings is an important part of the qualitative research process (p. 217), lending valuable insight and depth to the research. Finlay (1998) too, offers reflexivity as a means of turning the problem of researcher subjectivity in research into an opportunity. In this contested field, value and credibility of the current study were addressed as follows.

Value and credibility of the current study

The value of the study was considered in line with the feminist tradition of valuing women's accounts (Reinharz, 1992). Feminist research is also credited with a greater concern for women's experiences (Finch, 1999; Kong, Mahoney, & Plummer, 2002; Reinharz, 1992; Oakley, 1981) and, in this study, my personal feminist philosophy encouraged a particular type of conversational friendly interview, described above. The evolving interview format was based on an understanding of the participants' standing in the community and their vulnerability as new mothers. This approach offered access to the women's ideas and thoughts in their own words, valuing their unique accounts. Feminist research approaches also commonly focus on the everyday lives of women (Kvale, 1996, p. 73), which was the prime intent of this study. Sharing a cultural milieu was also seen as advantageous, in allowing access to the participants, a view shared by Wasserfall (1997). From my own experiences with childbearing women, particularly vulnerable primiparae over 35, I am convinced that this study would not have been possible if the researcher was other than female and of a similar age to participants.

In terms of supporting credibility and reducing the likelihood of flawed findings in this study, efforts were made to promote a faithful presentation of the experiences of new motherhood, as described by participants. Indeed, presentation of faithful description is central to credibility in qualitative research (Koch, 1998; Sandelowski, 1986) and confirmation of findings by returning transcripts to participants is prominently advised as a qualitative check (Cutliffe & McKenna, 1999; Emden, 1998). Member checking, staunchly advocated by Erlandson, Harris, Skipper and Allen (1993), is employed here. Although similar in many respects to returning transcripts to participants, member checking, for the purpose of this study, refers to the ongoing clarification of participant intent, as described below. The use of participants' own words in the findings is also seen as valuable and as likely to contribute to a faithful description (Cutliffe & McKenna, 1999; Emden, 1998; Erlandson et al., 1993). In the current study, each of these measures was employed.

Returning transcripts to the participants

Cutliffe and McKenna suggest that "if the emerging story has captured the essence of the phenomenon... under review, then the participants are likely to recognise themselves in it" (1999, pp. 378-379). In the final stage of data analysis of this study, an overview of themes was sent to each participant, as discussed earlier, and participant feedback and commentary were invited. Feedback indicated that the results closely matched the experiences of the career women, with many participants returning the sheets covered in ticks to represent the experiences they recognised. Others, while recognising some shared experiences, commented that their experiences were not quite so intense. Ideally, a second flow sheet should have represented differing experiences.

Member checking

Member checking is another method of promoting credibility of findings and Erlandson et al. (1993) are particularly vocal in their support. Sandelowski, however, urges caution and suggests that participants may not always be "in the best position to check the accuracy of an account, as they may have forgotten the information they provided or the manner in which it was provided" (1993, p. 6). For the current study, I particularly liked Sandelowski's (1993) view that ongoing member checking occurs throughout interviews, each time the interviewer seeks to clarify a statement or intent. In the current study, I frequently engaged in this level of checking and I would often repeat my understandings of a participant's account and seek her confirmation that I had 'got it right'. Similarly, I sought clarification of meanings that were unclear.

Use of the participants' own words

Use of the participants' own words provides another means of presenting faithful description and is commonly advised within texts. Indeed, Erlandson et al. (1993) have suggested that "thick description will bring the reader vicariously into the setting the researcher is describing" (p. 24) and this was the intent of the current study. Here, extensive use of data is employed and emergent themes are illustrated principally in the participants' words. In this way, the power of the women's words remains undiminished.

In the following section, the utility of audit trails for the purpose of this study and as a further measure of researcher transparency is considered.

Audit trail

Audit trails are highly recommended as a measure of researcher transparency and credibility of study findings (Koch, 1998; Speciale & Carpenter, 2003). Details of analytic decisions and themes arising from the data provide a trail which an independent researcher or auditor may follow. In this study, I have tracked my progress through data analysis and analytic decisions by means of memos and a journal. In this way, I kept track of thoughts and reflections and traced emerging thoughts and themes. While this was initiated to help me to track my emerging thoughts, it also provides a clear record of the analytic journey.

In the final section of this chapter, the participants are presented in terms of social demographics, in self-described groups. This categorisation is in keeping with the focus of social context for contemporary mothers.

Participants

Although, on the face of it, it would appear that the participants were a homogenous group, there were nonetheless some interesting demographic variations noted and the women were self-described as 'high-achieving' or 'really wanting a baby'. The groupings are ordered by the narratives participants offered and the self-categorisations they employed, particularly in relation to their motivation in having a baby at this stage of their lives and their reasons for postponement of pregnancy. There is, expectedly, a certain degree of overlap and I have tried to be faithful to the women's self descriptions.

Common to both groups of older mothers was the spectre of infertility that overhung their various experiences of postponement of pregnancy, unanticipated inability to conceive, fertility treatments and subsequent conception. Most described feeling that they were running out of time, even when no difficulty was experienced. Several viewed the pregnancy as 'last chance'.

In the ensuing table socio demographic characteristics of the various groups are displayed. Greater participant detail is then presented.

Group characteristics.

Career women over 35 years n = 16	Dream-come-true over 35 years n = 6	Young achievers approx 30 years n = 5
Age range 35-48 years	Age range 35-43 years	Age range 27-31years
Natural conception = 9	Natural conception = 3	Natural conception = 5
IVF = 5 Fertility treatment other than IVF = 2	IVF = 3 Fertility treatment other than IVF = 0	IVF = 0 Fertility treatment other than IVF = 0
Electively postponed childbearing	Did not electively postpone childbearing	3 unplanned pregnancies 2 planned
Considered work very important	Considered work less important than family	Considered work very important
Educated to tertiary level / Significant career investment	Educated to secondary level or below Limited career investment	Educated to tertiary level / Significant career investment
Professional / business occupations	Occupations mostly administrative / clerical	Professional / business occupations
1 set twins	1 set twins	No twins

Career women

In general, these women tended to be well-educated [tertiary degree or more] and were self-proclaimed 'high achievers' and 'perfectionists'. They included a doctor, a journalist, accountants, lawyers, businesswomen, an academic, computer specialists, a project manager, a teacher and a registered nurse. For the most part, they described approaching childbearing as a well delineated 'plan' and most had reached a certain level of career achievement prior to choosing to conceive. Some participants had been married or in a stable relationship for as long as 17 years and had postponed childbearing in pursuit of other goals / career plans. For some, the motivation for having a baby at this point in time was related to feeling that: 'time was running out'; or that now was the 'right time'. For two mothers, increasing dissatisfaction with work provided the trigger. A total of 16 mothers fitted this category. Of the seven women older than forty, five had required some degree of intervention to conceive. Of these five, all had taken significantly longer to conceive than anticipated.

Dream-come-true

In stark contrast to their more accomplished sisters, this group of women were less likely to have actively delayed childbearing and many had wanted a baby for quite some time. In general, they tended to be less well-educated and participated in occupations such as: hairdresser, receptionist and clerk. Their parturition plans had been thwarted by lack of a partner, divorce, reluctance in a partner or fertility difficulties. They tended to describe being 'really ready for a baby / aching for one' and, when their dreams were achieved, felt 'truly blessed'. There were also two women, who mostly fitted in this category due to their educational and work experiences, who had delayed pregnancy, one due to ill-health and one due to 'being scared'. A total of six women fitted this category. Again, the older members of this group (greater than 40 years) were more likely to have experienced unanticipated delays in conception.

Young Achievers

This group consisted of a small sample of younger women, aged approximately 30 years, recruited purposively on the basis of significant career investment. Interestingly, of the 5 women recruited, two had planned pregnancies for this time in their lives and the remaining three had unplanned pregnancies. For them, plans had included a postponement of childbearing to a later stage in their careers and the unplanned pregnancies created some difficulties, such as rearrangement of financial plans and living arrangements.

Summary

In this chapter, storytelling has been reviewed as the principal means by which individuals make sense of life events and the temporality of individual stories has been discussed. With this in mind, participant stories were considered a useful way to access the experience of mothering and the social context of women's lives for this study's participants. The particular methodology employed here was chosen as it permitted a valuing of individual's stories and recognised the part stories play in the social construction of self. This methodology was largely informed by Hardin's (2001) understanding of stories as 'nested within a background of broader social and cultural discourses' and thus was entirely congruent with the study's post-structural intent (p. 11). The researcher's feminist views have also contributed.

The sample has been presented in terms of size, recruitment criteria and strategies, and methodological decisions made during the course of this study and the justifications therein have been presented unequivocally. Data analysis has also been described through steps of transcription, reduction and thematic analysis. Issues of study credibility and value were then attended, as was the researcher's struggle to position herself within the research. Finally, the participants have been presented in three groups as a prelude to chapter 4.

In chapter 4, the 'project' is presented as the first stage in the temporal sequence of transition to motherhood. Within the 'project', maternal approach to mothering for the current participants is discussed together with the tendency to read and prepare extensively for impending motherhood.

CHAPTER 4
THE PROJECT

Tanya, an accountant, is 39 and has been married for 12 years, during which time she has studied and pursued her career. She had always planned to have children 'one day', but has waited for the right time both personally and professionally. Last year on Tanya's 38th birthday, she and Mark, her husband, decided that 2002 would be 'the year'. In preparation, Tanya has been on folic acid for 12 months and during this time has visited several maternity hospitals, a nutritionist and her GP for pre-pregnancy health checks. Happily, she and Mark conceive easily and since becoming pregnant Tanya has attended Yoga and 'preggi-bellies' exercise classes. She also has attended 3 different lots of pre-natal education classes in her quest for information and has bought all 24 books of the recommended reading lists from her various classes. Tanya and Mark have had many discussions on the way they will share child-raising tasks and have formulated plans to ensure the baby will fit into their life rather than 'changing everything' to accommodate the infant. They have been particularly concerned about 'sleeping issues' and this has been fuelled by stories of their friends' experiences. They have decided that the baby must get used to its own room from the beginning and have plans to 'establish a routine' as a priority. I first meet Tanya in the postnatal ward, surrounded by childcare manuals and in tears because it is all 'going wrong'.

In this study, 'the project' represents the first stage of transition to motherhood experiences for participants as elicited by the research question "What is the experience of first mothering for women over 35?" In general, transition to motherhood occurred for this study's participants in a temporally ordered sequence, commencing for many women well in advance of conception. High-achieving and successful women, in particular, applied a carefully constructed plan to conceiving under optimal conditions and invested considerable energy in 'doing it properly', that is, growing and birthing a baby. There was a tendency to approach childbearing as any other major project in the woman's life and the more professional women displayed a clearly defined trajectory of information seeking, decision making and planning. For these women, the 'project' was successfully completed with the birth of a healthy infant.

Overall, the 'project' involved a considerable amount of pre-pregnancy planning and discussion with the woman's partner and was largely informed by reading material and information gleaned from friends. Decisions around acceptable social behaviour and discipline of the child were made well in advance of the birth. Worries about 'being manipulated by the baby' and 'starting bad habits' featured largely in these discussions. Plans to establish a routine early and to pre-empt sleeping difficulties were also prominent, and seemed to be underwritten by an anxiety to perform well as a mother.

Despite common associations of older professional mothers as the purveyors of elaborate birth plans, this study found to the contrary and mothers here were less concerned with the birth experience than with a successful outcome.

In this chapter, the 'project' like approach favoured by study participants is discussed, through its three phases of: information seeking; planning and preparing, and finally, setting up the plan. Secondly, birth plans and classes, for the participants, are briefly discussed. Thirdly, career and work implications are examined, particularly with regard to work / pregnancy tensions as experienced by the participants. Finally, pregnancy and birth-related concerns, as articulated by the mothers at this stage, are discussed.

The project / 'doing it properly'

These women are educated, they are extremely well read, but they still want an answer, the baby is like a project and it's so uncontained ...

Cathy [M&CHN]

As Cathy, [M&CHN] identifies, having a baby was approached by many of the study mothers as a project. Following a decision to have a baby, there was a tendency, particularly among the career women, to approach childbearing as any other major project in their lives. The more professional women displayed a clearly defined trajectory of information seeking, planning and preparing and setting up the plan, which began long before conception and continued throughout the pregnancy. Pre-pregnancy reading focused on preparing the body for pregnancy and optimising chances of conception. Considerable attention was given to 'being as well informed as possible about the process' of pregnancy and birth. In this chapter, the project steps are dealt with sequentially, although information gathering and planning continued in tandem throughout most of the pregnancy and early stages of mothering.

Information seeking

The quest for information described by career women and to a lesser extent young-achievers, in this study, was quite extensive. Several women had read as many as twelve pregnancy guides and popular works. Some had read several more. One woman, who had attended three different lots of pre-natal education classes, had read all eight recommended titles on class reading lists, a total of twenty-four texts. For several of the participants, this was a normal work strategy. Before commencing any new work-related project, particularly an important one, the women would research and read extensively, approaching the new situation as well-informed as possible. For these women it made sense to research childbearing in a similar fashion. Sally [career woman] explains:

I found it a challenge, like everything I take on ... a challenge, and like whatever I do ... I research it then find out what I have to do and put it all together and do it!

For Gayle [career woman], concerns about the 'success' of her new project drove her quest for information:

If this thing is going to work we're going to have to, we're going to have to make sure it's a success ...

In general, although the majority of the career women researched childbearing, pregnancy and mothering extensively, there was a recognition that extensive knowledge might prove anxiety provoking. Here, Harriet [career woman] explains feeling it important to be as well informed as possible, but was aware that 'knowing too much' might be a cause for concern:

That was very important for me, to be as knowledgeable as I could be about the process that my body was going through. I did read a lot ... on[sic]the same token I think over-information can be a mistake ... you think you've got everything, every condition under the sun ...

Type of information

One interesting point was the type of information these women sought and the marked difference between the information required by the more accomplished women, compared to dream-come-true mothers. Career women were often dismissive of popular reading material, showing a clear preference for information of a medical / scientific / nursing bent. Several women trawled the Internet for more extensive information when dissatisfied with that provided by doctors or midwives. Here, Margaret [career woman] describes her attitude to reading material:

Well, we read a lot of books, ... I had about 6 or 7 really good reference books on pregnancy ... in the middle I think John got bored and he stopped reading and I kept reading them all madly ... some of the books are really terrific, we had a couple of really authoritative ones, one from the Royal Women's' [hospital] in Sydney, I think it was written by obstetricians and nurses ...

Rosie [career woman] was dismissive of 'silly stuff' presented in popular literature:

I read lots, the pamphlets from the hospital and stuff, and Kaz, Kaz? [Kaz Cooke] My friend had given me ... sometimes I was quite serious and I wanted to get down to business and they were going on and on, ... cut to the core with the silly stuff!

Specific information quests

Each new or unanticipated event sparked additional information-seeking quests for a percentage of the well-educated older mothers. For example, the discovery of the fetus in a breech position would often result in the mother reading extensively on percentages of fetuses presenting as breech, likely causes of this presentation and the success rates of external cephalic version[16]. Elizabeth, an academic, presents a poignant example. The discovery of a two-vessel cord [instead of the more usual three vessel cord] on ultrasound initiated an impressive information quest, both in Australia and overseas, as she found it difficult to access the depth of information she required:

Trying to get the information I needed was difficult! ... I felt that every time they told about something that I had, like the one artery [in the cord] that was a different branch of research that I couldn't get from them [midwives]. I think that was a little frustrating, because I'm somebody who'd liked to research ... but when I found one of these problems I would try to research [in the USA]. It was only in American books that I found reference to it ... [2 vessel cord]

One element of extensive information searching related to an issue of trust, and the more accomplished women endorsed an attitude of 'if I do it myself I know it is done', that most probably served them well in their working lives. Several described a mistrust of the doctor's / midwife's knowledge, or a failure to answer questions to their satisfaction, as inspiring personal quests for expert or more in-depth opinion. Jane [career woman] explains:

---

[16] manually turning a baby presenting by the breech in order to facilitate normal vaginal delivery

70

I looked up a lot on folic acid because I was a bit worried that I was having too little ... and my doctor particularly ... I'd ask him something and it'd be a very quick answer! I wanted to discuss all sorts of issues. I bought a lot of books and read them, but sometimes I looked for more information, like I would read something and [think] 'Oh that's interesting, but didn't give me enough' and I'd tend to look up more on the internet or look for another book ... the gynaecologist was far too dismissive for my liking! So I would often leave there feeling like I didn't get my questions answered ... he would brush me off and I found that really frustrating.

Although most career women employed extensive information gathering in a bid to be well informed, a smaller percentage of the mothers in this group found the more clinical books frightening and difficult to comprehend. Jane [career woman] felt it was important to be well informed, but was more focused on how others had coped and found clinical tomes difficult to deal with:

I think probably ... as soon as I found out I was pregnant I wanted information, I wanted to know how other people coped! I was well aware there were decisions to make ... so I wanted to know how other people coped with it, I suppose, and also experience is the best guide so having no experience [I] sought out other people's experiences to see how they coped ... there's so many books out there, a lot of people gave me other books to read, but[when] I started to read it [sic] and it was so technical and clinical and I just thought 'ooh, can't cope.'

Dream-come-true group

In contrast, women from the dream-come-true group were less concerned about information gathering and showed, in general, a preference for more humorous books or relied on a single book for their information needs. After carefully selecting their text, they describe reading and re-reading sections on a need-to-know basis, reading first trimester information when newly pregnant and moving forward as the pregnancy advanced. Another interesting variation among this group was the tendency to purchase reading material only after becoming pregnant, rather than research pre-pregnancy information such as folic acid. Annie [dream-come-true] describes meeting her information needs:

71

When I first fell pregnant, I went and bought a book, because I just had no idea what to do, no idea ... now that someone's told me that I'm pregnant, it was like 'what do I do'? Do I stop eating certain foods? Do I have to eat anything different? So I went and bought a book, I looked through all the books in the bookstore and picked out the one that I thought was going to be enough, and just read that. One day I had pains right down the side, and I thought 'that's a bit strange' and went to the book, 21 weeks or whatever, and it said 'you might feel pains down the side' and it was just bizarre, everything that was happening was in there ...

Young-achievers

Young-achievers tended to be extremely busy getting their lives in order, organising finances, maternity leave and sometimes alternate accommodation during pregnancy. Pregnancy was unplanned for all but two mothers in this group. Two of the women had had difficulty booking into the hospital of their choice and had spent quite some time finding an obstetrician to care for them. Of the women with planned pregnancies, information gathering was attended in a manner reminiscent of career women. Anita [young achiever] found the information she received from the hospital and health centre insufficient for her needs. However, more advanced reading proved anxiety provoking:

I mean I've gone and read through a lot of pamphlets and information I've received from the hospital ... they're all dribs and drabs, they don't really answer the question that you're looking for ... I'd be reading about the low placenta thing, and what's the other one called when your blood pressure is high ... I was reading through that and I'd think maybe I've got that, got something towards the end.

The younger women in general, tended not to display the same level of concern around the pregnancy, and if anything tended to be pragmatic in their approach. Melanie [young achiever] a doctor working in an acute facility, focused on normalising pregnancy, and had a very down-to-earth approach:

I've never been one of those people to sit and think 'oh my gosh! The miracle of life and all that, it was like OK the baby's growing, that's good, that's fine, and I had a couple of books that I got that he [husband] could read ...

Pregnancy-related information gathering, *per se*, is not abundantly addressed within the literature. There is however, a clearly demonstrated trend among older, middle-class, educated mothers, to prepare for mothering through extensive reading and information searching (Deutsch, Brooks-Gunn, Fleming, Ruble & Stangor, 1988; Gottesman, 1992; Mercer, 1986; Viau, Padula & Eddy, 2002). In this study, many mothers read avidly, conducted Internet searches and recruited information from doctors' surgeries and hospitals. Similarly, Viau et al. (2002), found that pregnant women over 35 were "pro-active healthcare seekers" accessing information from a wide variety of sources to meet their individual needs (p. 328). Again, similar to the findings of this study, increased maternal awareness of fetal and infant risks among older first-time mothers, is found within the literature (Dobrzykowski & Stern, 2003; Meisenhelder & Meservey, 1987), and this group of mothers are identified as the group most likely to attend childbirth education classes (Cliff & Deery, 1997; Lu, Prentice, Yu, Inkelas, Lange & Halfon, 2003).

Overall, increasing consumer confidence and awareness of one's rights, tend to result in individuals requesting additional information in a whole variety of situations, and this trend is increasingly obvious among maternity patients. Singh, Newburn, Smith and Wiggins (2002), who conducted a widespread survey of pregnant British women

(n = 702), across a range of socio-economic groupings, found that two thirds of the respondents would have liked more pregnancy-related information, while Emmanuel, Creedy and Fraser (2001) found that pre-natal preparation, in general, did not meet pregnant women's educational needs.

Planning and preparing

Planning and preparing occurred throughout the entire project and the principal emphasis was on 'getting it right' and 'doing it properly'. Career women and to a lesser extent young-achievers, invested considerable time in preparing mentally and physically for pregnancy and birth. Prior to pregnancy, this involved getting 'really healthy', visiting doctors and nutritionists and deciding on pregnancy and delivery care options. This phase went hand-in-hand with information gathering and involved visiting hospitals and checking out maternity services. Several career women described calling hospitals for lists of practicing obstetricians and possible recommendations and checking out facilities such as neonatal intensive care units and advanced services. Women of the dream-come-true group had, in general, a more pragmatic approach to pregnancy care and tended to rely on the recommendations of family and friends. Young-achievers endorsed an approach that was located somewhere between the two. Maximising health status prior to conception was a strategy employed by all three groups. Jane's

73

[career woman] careful attention to diet and physical preparation commenced before conception and continued throughout pregnancy. However, she also visited a physician to have her blood pressure checked although it had not previously troubled her, as she knew from her reading that elevated blood pressure was frequently associated with older maternity. She explains:

I was very careful! I went and spoke to a dietician and ... never drank so much milk! I've never drunk or smoked, so, I've been lucky in that regard, but I did want to make sure that at least my diet was giving him the right things. We went to lots of doctors to make sure I did everything right. I went to a blood pressure specialist, to make sure my blood pressure did not get out of hand, I mean, it had not been a problem, but we thought that it was a possibility ...

Jeanne [dream-come-true] describes attending her doctor for a pre-pregnancy health check:

First of all I did things like well I made sure that my Rubella was all right, so the physical medical side of it was OK. I'd started ... I'd already started to take Folic acid long before I got pregnant and just taking multivitamins, just to be sure, won't hurt ...

Sharon's [young achiever] careful preparation included ceasing the contraceptive pill six months prior, taking folate and making efforts to be fit and healthy, in order to give her baby the best possible start:

The plan was to go away and have a big holiday and to come back and start trying ... so we came back, went off the pill and went off for 6 months before we started trying, did the ... prepare your body and take the folate and whatever ... so I wanted to give her the best start you could possibly ...

Once pregnant, most of the study participants made efforts to remain healthy and well. The most extravagant efforts were again concentrated among the more highly accomplished women, who additionally may have had more scope related to higher income levels. Gayle [career woman] continued to swim and attend yoga sessions until late in pregnancy, using yoga to assist with the discomforts of advanced pregnancy:

As for preparing me, body-wise, I just kept up doing my swimming ... I kept up my fitness in general, I've always done lots of swimming ... until I got to the point where I could hardly do it, when my legs were so swollen ... When the legs started to swell up I started to get worried and up until that time I was doing yoga ...

Rachel [career woman] concentrated on eating well and exercising and attended a variety of specialised pregnancy exercise classes:

I ate really well and those sorts of things, ... Ate well, always slept fairly well, alcohol, just cut down on that, did exercise, but then I usually do anyway! I went to preggi-belly classes, exercise classes, water aerobic classes and that sort of thing ...

Within the literature, maternal education, socio-economic status and older maternal age at first birth are all linked to greater attention to health choices (Berkowitz et al., 1993; Berryman et al., 1999; Ventura, 1989) and, similar to the findings of this study, greatest effort seems to be concentrated among the most highly-educated women (Berkowitz et al., 1993; Berryman et al., 1999). Maternal education is also linked to a host of other health related factors, such as greater access to health care (Morrison et al., 1989; Raum et al., 2001) and reduced rates of smoking (Berkowitz et al., 1993; Ventura, 1989).

Pregnancy or baby

For women of the dream-come-true group, much of the pre-natal time was spent thinking and wondering about the **baby** rather than the **pregnancy,** which is strikingly different from the approach employed by the more accomplished women, who tended to concentrate on 'doing it [the pregnancy] properly'. For dream-come-true mothers, there was a limited emphasis on physical preparation prior to conception, although each of the women made considerable effort to 'do the right thing' during pregnancy, regarding diet and avoidance of alcohol and cigarettes. Annie, [dream-come-true] for example, was particularly concerned about diet and inhaling cigarette smoke:

I worried about what I was doing and how I was eating and how I was running my life and how it was affecting her ... I was worried about people smoking around me because I know passive smoking is bad, went off your [sic] junk food and everything ...

Choosing a hospital

Choosing a hospital was an important consideration for each of the mothers participating in this study, as was the choice of obstetrician or care model. Differences are however noted in the women's approach to decision making in this area, with the more professional women tending to shop around and rely on personal impressions gleaned from hospital visits and GP[17] recommendations. Many spoke of choosing venues where 'all the facilities' were available. Dream-come-true mothers tended to rely more on the recommendations of friends and family and would often refer to comments relating to the doctor's personality. Annie [dream-come-true] for example, chose her doctor on the recommendation of her friend:

> *My friend thought he was lovely and so approachable ...*

This tendency may also reflect sociological differences among the groups, where older primiparous women are more likely to live some distance from family and may not have any close friends or peers with young children (Ambler Walter, 1986; Cook, 1993) and thus may have to rely on different information sources. For many of the career women in this study, choice of hospital often related to 'risk management strategies'. Harriet [career woman] explains:

> *It was very important to me to have a really good doctor and that was, as soon as I realised I was pregnant which was 2 days after my period was due, I went to the GP and booked in to my doctor and everything, that was really important to me ... I chose a hospital where there was all, ... everything ... all the medical... [neonatal intensive care facilities]*

For Gayle [career woman] choosing a hospital also included such considerations as emergency back-up facilities:

> *I wanted to go somewhere where they could do an emergency section, just in case and I thought at my age and everything, I think I'd prefer to go there ...*

---

[17] general practitioner or local doctor

76

Of the seven women availing of fertility treatments to conceive, choice of hospital was never a major consideration, they simply had not considered delivering anywhere other than the tertiary level hospital where they had received treatment, though their pregnancies were considered essentially normal.

In the following section, birth plans and pre-natal classes, as consistent with maternal preparation, are discussed.

Birth plans

Despite a common perception of first-time mothers over 35 as the purveyors of elaborate birth plans, this was not borne out in the current study. Many participants, particularly those mothers who had experienced some difficulty conceiving, were less interested in birth plans and maternal empowerment than in delivering the infant safely. Anthea [career woman] explains her attitude:

I'd already agreed with the obstetrician 'just do whatever you've got to do. That's your department! Yeah and you just tell me what to do, just don't leave me in the dark ... like prior to the labour, I'd said to him 'what about a birth plan?' Because the group were talking about a birth plan, but I'm not into that 'load of crock', so ... I asked him and he said 'no, I'm not into any of that' ... he said exactly what I wanted to hear!

In contrast, a small number of the dream-come-true group subscribed to the 'romantic birth' notion. This notion appears to be largely co-constructed within social discourses, including articles in women's magazines and childbirth education classes and to a certain extent the industry that markets such products as aromatherapy candles. Within this view, birth is often portrayed as the crowning achievement of a woman's life (Kaplan, 1992; Marshall, 1991) and as a wonderful shared experience for her partner. Planning involves classical music choices, aromatherapy and relaxing techniques and, as one critic caustically suggested, the infant is expected to float out on a cloud of aromatherapy. Jennifer [dream-come-true] had envisaged a romantic birth and had gone to considerable effort to 'create the mood' but was nonetheless ill prepared for the pain of labour:

What I was prepared for was the fairytale, I had the gorgeous nighties, I had everything happening, I thought I was going to sit up there with the nails painted, with the make-up, everything ... but what happened was that she was 41 weeks ... I had to be induced, I went in that afternoon ... I thought they'll induce me, I'll get a few contractions, pain, pain, like a period pain but I'll cope, I can breathe through it ... And what actually happened was that they put the gel and it immediately took effect .... They said go for a walk, I got up and I was crippled and Ian was looking at me, [like]... you're making this up!

Indeed, among this study's participants and especially among older mothers, perceptions of increased pregnancy risk and fetal / infant vulnerability were more likely to influence decisions around birth than any other consideration.

Pre-natal classes

All but one of the study participants attended pre-natal education classes, similar to literature findings of greater attendance among primigravid women (Cliff & Deery, 1997; Lu et al. 2003). Most enjoyed the classes and valued the interaction with other expectant parents. Career women and young-achievers however, tended to be more practically focused and were often disappointed with birthing classes' scant reference to postpartum care of the infant. Many were so well read that there was no new information available at the classes. Still others had attended primarily for the benefit of their spouses' education.

Kerri [career woman], had a very pragmatic approach, probably largely informed by her experiences as a critical care nurse:

I didn't get a real lot out of the classes, probably because I had the wrong expectations, I thought they would teach you a lot more practical things. I thought they would teach you how to change a nappy ... they talked a lot more about things that I thought were a bit airy fairy, like what music you wanted in the labour ward and what aromatherapy. That was not for me ... I was not planning on any of that anyway, I was just straight down the line, just get it over and done with!

The experiences of young-achievers were similar to the career women, in that they tended to be well read and often attended prenatal classes largely for their spouses' benefit. Their approach too, tended to be practically focused with little emphasis on 'romantic' birth.

For Kim [young achiever], attending a weekend workshop was a matter of choosing to 'get it over and done with', as she was already well versed in delivery expectations. Her principal interest related to informing and involving her husband and she felt compassion for the 'poor woman' [over 35] who was taking notes:

> *We could've gone to the 2 hours a week, but when there was the option of the Sunday, I thought no, get it over and done with, I knew the stages of labour and I know all the routine stuff ... I think it was good for him [husband] to see the forceps and the suction cap ... and tears and episiotomies ... one poor woman I felt really sorry for her, she took about 15 pages of notes over the day ... she said she had never had had any contact with a baby and David said to me 'do I need to be writing any thing down? [I said] Naw, we'll get through this ...*

Interestingly, despite elaborate preparation in other areas, several of the career women describe an almost paralysing inability to prepare materially for the infant.

Inability to prepare

Worries about the health of the baby often contributed to anxiety and an inability to prepare in any material sense for taking the infant home and this trend was seen almost exclusively among the career women of this study. This manifested in a reluctance to prepare a room or buy items such as a cot or a pram. Although common among career women, this attitude was often in stark contrast to other members of birthing classes. Harriet explains:

> *It was quite funny when we went to the pre-natal classes, everyone else in the room would say we've done this and we've done that ... we'd done nothing!... and Simon's mother kept saying we needed to do something, she kept on saying 'you've got the room ready, you've packed your bag? We got the pram about a few weeks before actually ... Well, the reason we didn't get round to it was 1. something could go wrong and even when we bought the pram and the car seat I said to Simon, 'keep the receipts in case we have to take them back' in case it's a stillborn, or anything like that. You know, the pessimistic attitude. It was a really, it was a big thing, I didn't want to get anything even out of the box ...*

In contrast, dream-come-true mothers were more likely to have a 'nursery' set up, long in advance of the birth. Many went to great lengths to create a particular 'look'. Janet explains her preparation:

My mother took me shopping, once I got past 12 weeks, we did lots of shopping, we've got a family antique bassinet, so my husband resprayed all that and we got a new mattress, a new net for the crook ...

Lack of engagement

Several of the mothers, again principally career women, described a tendency to feel removed from the pregnancy and employed strategies such as keeping busy to prevent negative thoughts from intruding. Others described not allowing themselves to look forward to this much-wanted birth and this tendency seems to relate to an inability to prepare for the baby, as described above. Abigail [career woman] explains:

I had not allowed myself ... to really look forward to it [the birth] ... I was so afraid and when I look back now to what I was like in the last 3 months of the pregnancy ... I was very, very scared about whether that baby was going to be OK!

In contrast, 'dream-come-true' mothers spent a considerable amount of time thinking about the baby they carried and often described knowing the baby well, while career women seldom visualised or dreamt about of the infant. Sally [career woman] explains:

A lot of women, a lot of my friends said that to me, have you dreamt about them [twins] but I haven't ... I was beginning to worry because everyone was saying have you been dreaming about them and I'd say no and I thought there's something wrong with me ...

Whereas Annie [dream-come-true] describes feeling 'very maternal' and here discusses her baby's hiccups:

We were sitting on the couch and the baby was jumping and jumping and I realised it's got hiccups ... and I was thinking 'oh the poor thing' I felt really really sorry for it! [patting her tummy] but the hiccup thing, here I go already, I'll be hopeless! It was really bizarre! It really was! I'm starting to feel very maternal!

80

Inability to prepare / lack of engagement / implications for early adjustment

In addition to a reluctance to prepare materially for the infant's homecoming, several career women also described deliberately holding in abeyance any thoughts they may have had about the baby, or how it might feel to be a mother. This attitude related to concerns that 'something might happen', meaning principally that the infant might not survive, and it seems likely that this lack of engagement with the pregnancy may later impact on the women's maternity experiences. Indeed, within the literature, engagement with the pregnancy has been frequently considered an important step in maternal identity acquisition (Cohen, 1979; Rubin 1967a, 1967b, 1984) and pregnancy is often discussed as a time of psychological preparation for mothering (Rossi, 1968; Rubin, 1984; Smith, 1999). The mother's acceptance of her pregnancy and attachment to the fetus are seen as important markers for future positive maternal adjustment (Gottesman, 1992; Leifer, 1980; Mercer, 1986; Muller, 1996; Sherehefsky & Yarrow, 1973). Indeed, Cohen (1979) considered lack of pregnancy engagement as predictive of later problems with mothering.

Additionally, several authors discuss early visualisation of oneself as a mother, as an important step in taking on the maternal role (Leifer, 1980; Rubin, 1984; Sherehefsky & Yarrow, 1973) and psychologist Myra Leifer (1980) found that prospective mothers in her study became increasingly keen, as pregnancy advanced, to be around mothers and children. Furthermore, Leifer suggested that expectant mothers often mentally tried out observed mothering techniques (p. 82) as they prepared psychologically for mothering. Rubin (1984) meanwhile, described a process where the prospective mother dreamt of, and imagined herself in the role of mother, envisaging the relationship she would share with her infant. Although Rubin's work bears the mark of 1950s/1960s American mothering, it nonetheless forms a useful comparison for framing the experiences of contemporary women. For Rubin, maternal role attainment commenced during pregnancy, with the pregnant woman's idealisation of herself as a mother being an important step in this process, a finding supported by Leifer.

In this study, several mothers appeared to miss out on this stage of idealisation of self as a mother during pregnancy, which may in turn be linked to a slower-than-usual attainment of maternal role, though the dearth of comparative literature makes direct comparison difficult. This later transition is discussed in greater detail in subsequent chapters. Interestingly, later maternal role attainment was not seen among dream-come-true mothers in this study and, indeed, these women appeared to form an emotional attachment to the fetus early in the pregnancy and to visualise and fondly refer to the baby by nickname. Mothers of this group described 'knowing' their infant well in advance of birth and would discuss understanding the infant's sleep / wake cycles from 'when he/she was inside me'.

81

Setting up a plan

Formulating and setting up the plan was the final stage of the project for study participants and involved two major areas of attention: socialisation of the infant to fit within the parents' lives and setting up home and work to allow for time with the infant. These two sub-themes are discussed in the following section.

Socialisation of the infant

In this study, career women showed particular interest in the socialisation of the infant, with many of the women having very clear ideas on how they would like their infant to behave. A considerable focus was on having the baby 'fit' into their lives, rather than 'changing everything around' to accommodate the baby. Considerations included continuing to play sport, dine out and travel. This stage involved multiple discussions with the woman's partner and decisions around acceptable social behaviour and discipline were made well in advance of the birth. These decisions were largely informed by friends' negative experiences of parenting. Worries about 'being manipulated by the baby' and 'starting bad habits' dominated these discussions. Plans to establish a routine early and to pre-empt sleeping difficulties are also prominent. Concerns about the spousal relationship also arose, with many women discussing and planning to have 'couple time', or 'our time' as well as caring for an infant. For Rachel, [career woman] it was important that the baby did not entirely disrupt the life she and her husband had built together, in their 10 years of marriage:

> *In planning to have a baby ... Kel and I are both fairly social people, we're very active people and I was just concerned that a baby would change all those things that we made, again, we sat down and discussed it numerous times, we both agreed that a baby was not going to totally dictate what we were going to do! That it would have to fit in with us as well, to fit in with our lifestyle...*

Rachel's principal concerns centred on being manipulated by her infant and she was convinced of a limited opportunity to develop 'good routines'. She was determined that she would not allow this to happen:

I have a fear that this tiny cute looking little person is going to dictate our lives totally and that can't happen. I heard all these stories ... the little I know about babies, it could be the start of him being a control freak!

Several mothers had pre-decided how they would mother, based on mothering strategies they had observed and liked in other mothers and would thus like to adopt. Anthea's [career woman] views were informed by watching her sisters parenting and concerns to pre-empt 'bad' behaviour. Here, she expresses worries about 'starting bad habits', particularly around sleeping:

I think this is probably being older and wiser, you've seen a lot, seen for example, of my 2 sisters one of them was a real quiet fusspot and the other one really was not ... and I thought if anything I'll be more like her as a mother. You see things in other people that you admire, you know ... I don't want to start bad habits, that's the other thing I'm conscious of, I've had friends that have [said] 'oh, he'll only settle in the sling, you don't need that, I mean, you'd get nothing done around the house because you're holding someone...

Indeed, several mothers were extremely concerned about instilling good sleep patterns in their infants and many had planned long in advance of birth, the strategies they would employ to ensure a full night's sleep. This finding is particularly marked among mothers who planned an early or full-time return to work. Gayle [career woman] who was returning to full-time academia, was keen to set up a routine early. Ensuring the baby slept was a major issue:

I have a friend, who's got a baby, who's a year old and I get all sorts of advice from her, she had all sorts of problems, sleeping and everything and she warned me don't do all the mistakes I made [sic] and think about what you're doing ... we had to get her into this routine coz I had to go back to work and she would have to behave at childcare, I know there are children there that have to be held to sleep, that's my greatest fear!

In contrast, mothers from the dream-come-true group tended not to make elaborate plans about routines or disciplining the infant. They also seemed less concerned with setting up bad habits or being manipulated by the baby. This may in part relate to plans to retire from work, or remain at home during at least the baby's first year. Overall, there seemed to be less urgency attached to having a 'manageable' plan. Janet [dream-come-true] explains:

I'm not afraid of spoiling her or anything like that ... you can't listen to everyone telling you do this or do that...

Annie [dream-come-true] decides to just 'go with the flow':

I didn't really have a lot of expectations really, ... I took things as they came I think I looked at it like that from the start laughter, I thought I'd be in for some shocks, but that's the way I do a lot of things, I go along ... I just go with the flow...

Young-achievers tended to be located somewhere between the two groups and the majority had planned an early return to full-time work. Nonetheless, there was an attitude of 'just dealing with it' expressed by these women. Kim [young-achiever] explains:

We didn't actually decide to have a baby, he just happened, so we would have actually planned it for another ... down the track ... I mean you can't send him back where he came from ... yeh but you just go with the flow and if you plan something and it doesn't happen well, so be it...

Setting up work and home

For many career women, this stage of the plan was the culmination of perhaps five to ten years of advance planning and may have included scaling back the family business or relocating the office to work from home. For others it included the purchase of a home or accommodation suited to raising a family. Some career women had just acquired a home, despite being married for as long as 8-17 years. This was sometimes related to work associated moves, with one woman moving 10 times in 12 years. Feeling a need to settle and establish ties had a bearing on these choices. Some participants had just re-established homes in their second marriages. In addition to setting up home, setting up work was also a major consideration with several women relocating office and scaling back consultancies or businesses. An important component of relocation plans was to allow for time with the baby. Margaret [career woman] describes how purchasing a home set the scene for a family:

84

Also buying a house down here (suburbs), like that it's a little bit villagey like, the beach and the piers there and that's partly thinking 'oh we can have a family, this is a nice place to be'...

Making time for partner

Making time for the woman's partner featured into the plans of most of the participants, driven by concerns that the intimate relationship might suffer, and this tendency was most marked among older mothers, irrespective of educational status. Kelly [career woman] and Gayle explain:

I think my main concern, even though I didn't think I'd do it, but hearing about how the mother and the baby have such bonding and the husband feeling sort of left out. We kept saying we've gotta make time for ourselves...

Gayle [career woman]:

That's another thing, we thought all that out and we were worried about the fact that our previously good relationship would be affected, it may well be, it's early days yet!

Young-achievers showed some similarities to career women, in terms of planning and preparing and trying to pre-empt relationship deterioration, but in general tended to be more accepting of the changes a baby might bring. Sharon [young achiever] explains:

I guess we were emotionally together, we were very much together and we were happy there weren't any kinks in our relationship, that was important to us, we could then cope with another person in our lives ... a close friend said 'what are you going to do? And I said what do you mean? ' but you won't be able to pop down the street, she'll be with you! it'll be such a hassle!... She was just sort of saying that your whole life was going to change and it was going to be this momentous sort of thing, ... but when you plan to have a child you think that that's what's going to happen ... And you just accept that it's just the next stage of your life...

In addition to domestic plans to accommodate the infant, participants in this study often spoke of making employment-related plans. Indeed, it was clear that work occupied a central position in the lives of many participants and this centrality impacted on the women's subsequent maternal experiences.

Work and pregnancy

In this final chapter section, career and work implications are addressed. At pregnancy onset, all but one of the participants were employed and for many, again particularly career women, work had been an important part of their lives for some considerable time. For young-achievers, work was also very important and all had plans to resume work in the near future. For women of the dream-come-true group, work occupied a position of lesser importance than did current childbearing and child-raising plans. Four sub-themes related to work present at this stage of this study. They are: plans to accommodate family and work; work / pregnancy tensions; social expectations around work and mothering, and finally, not wanting to waste time.

Plans to accommodate family and work

Here, several career women planned to scale back their consultancy / businesses and to keep things 'ticking over' during child raising. For Anthea, Jane, Cassie and Sally this meant moving the office home and working 1-4 days a week from home. Abigail and Jane were in a position to do contract / free-lance work at home and were thus able to dictate the hours they worked. Others like Margaret and Kerri planned to return to part-time work. The remaining eight career women planned to resume full-time work. Anthea [career woman] explains her choices:

> *I had this shop and I thought we're going to start a family, we were trying at that stage so I actually moved it all home and set up the front room, with the plan being that I could have the children and keep the business going as a part-time concern.*

Jane [career woman] meanwhile, had built up a client profile during her many years as a senior accountant and during pregnancy set up a home office planning to continue with contract work:

So we set about to plan how we'd do it, like with work and have a child and the best way to do it was to work from home and I had a lot of contacts so I was able to start working, doing contract work ... [I] could mould it around having a child and having the business...

Several of the career women felt that they would be unable to continue to work at the job they previously held, due to long hours, unreasonable expectations around overtime or perceived levels of stress. Margaret explains:

I knew I couldn't have that career that I had before, it was not 9-5, it was 9-9, that seemed to be the primary thing, I wanted to be able to make enough time for a child...

For these women, the decision to return to part-time work or to pass up on career advancement opportunities was not always without a struggle. Kirsten's account is perhaps a little wistful:

And I suppose that you do give away career opportunities and even during the time that I was pregnant a few job opportunities came up that would've been perfect for me and I thought 'Oh well! The job that I have at the moment, I know is not a job you could have with a baby. I've seen someone else try to do it and it was really hard...

Work-related tensions

As discussed in chapter 3, maternal employment presents throughout this study as an interweaving thread and, at this juncture, it presents in terms of work / pregnancy tensions. For some of this study's participants, again particularly career women, leaving work even temporarily was a huge wrench and many described feeling torn between their various responsibilities. For most, there was an emphasis on completing tasks prior to taking maternity leave. The principal sub-themes then, presenting during the 'project' stage of this study and relating to work tensions were: a reluctance to tell colleagues; organising my own replacement; late commencement of maternity leave; not wanting to waste time and finally, social expectations around maternity leave. As this trend of work-related tensions was seen almost exclusively among the career-women only their accounts are presented here.

Reluctance to tell colleagues

Several women had had a prolonged wait for the 'right time' to have a baby, and for them, pregnancy represented the culmination of many years of planning. Yet, they spoke of a reluctance to tell their colleagues of the pregnancy until it was well advanced. This tendency seemed to relate to "not wanting to be seen in a different light", as Harriet explains:

> *I didn't tell any one, I didn't tell work until I was 23 weeks pregnant, one reason was that I didn't want people to see me in a different light at work ... there is [a] status attached to pregnancy, and 'oh, she can't do her job as well now' etc. etc.*

Organising my own replacement

An emphasis on the completion of important tasks prior to leaving was common and some women went to extraordinary lengths to organise their own replacements and were concerned about 'letting work down'. Some, like Harriet were aware that although she was legally entitled to return to her position, and indeed she planned to, nonetheless, she was aware that the incumbent/s in her position might expect to keep that position:

> *I wanted to get my project pretty much completed and sorted ... I did all my planning well in advance so I planned for when I left ... and then you've also got that whole replacement issue, and I found replacements for me, we found 4 people, we broke my job up to 4 and I actually found the replacements in advance ... then you have the guilt that if you go back that they lose their position...*

Laura continued to put in long days until the end of her pregnancy, despite her concerns about the 'fragility' of her IVF pregnancy and about her ability to carry to term. Her motivation was to arrange strategies for her absence:

> *I worked until 38 weeks, at the end of that, and I was still doing like a 10 hour day, at the end, like, I just want to stop now, that's why I was there for so long and worked so hard, because I was trying to put all the stuff in place so that it would be OK.*

Late commencement of maternity leave

For a number of the participants, particularly those employed in a position of seniority, late commencement of maternity leave was *de rigueur*. Some commenced maternity leave only in the week preceding their due date, sometimes against medical advice. One woman finished work only on the day of her scheduled induction of labour for elevated blood pressure, taking a taxi from work to the hospital. Gayle [career woman] explains:

> *On Tuesday I started to get protein in the urine, he said to me 'You're going in [to hospital] tonight' and I was supposed to go in that night and I got in there and I went into a 4 bed ward, and I said 'I can't stay here ... I just thought, I think I'd be better off at home tonight. I'm only in here to be observed ... Then I was supposed to come back in and I was not supposed to go to work the next day but I went in and I was there until 4 'o clock ... I had to go and hand over to the new girl ... Geoff [obstetrician] had been telling me about 3 weeks before that I had to leave and I said 'Geoff, I can't leave, I have to run maternity leave from the day it happens and secondly, I said I've got to hand over to the person ... in fact I went home at 4! I got in a cab and I was back at 5 and everyone was saying you're late he's going to induce you in half an hour.*

Not wanting to waste time

Several of the women in both the career women and young-achievers groups were keen not to 'waste time' by commencing maternity leave too early. Still others used their maternity leave 'productively' to finish study or complete a thesis, and to keep up with professional development plans. Kerri [career woman] didn't like the idea of wasting time on leave prior to giving birth. Here she explains her attitude:

> *I didn't want to be 2 weeks late and be thinking 'oh, now I'm hanging around' so I tried not to think about it happening...*

Harriet [career woman], used her maternity leave productively to complete her masters thesis:

> *I wanted to finish the Masters ... I'm quite happy to have a subject to complete next year, to do on my maternity leave, it means I won't lapse in my professional development...*

Torn between conflicting responsibilities

In general, the more career orientated women tended to work longer hours and take later maternity leave.

Many felt torn between their responsibilities to work, family and the growing fetus. Laura [career woman] explains:

> *I think also ... I'm sure a lot of the other women who were sort of professional, working as well feel that responsibility there as well, as well as to the baby you're carrying, as well as to the husband at home who's sitting there waiting for you to come home at 8 o'clock.*

Social expectations around working

Many women described an awareness of societal expectations that the baby's needs should be deemed more important and worthy than the woman's ongoing career, which created a tension around returning to work, particularly full-time work. Harriet [career woman] explains:

> *There's an underlying assumption that you won't come back ... I did say to one woman something about ... I said I've put about 15 years into my career and I'll probably come back half way through the year, next year, and she said that's about the amount of time I put into my daughter!... But it was the idea, because that was the perception too, that if you do go back you're doing the wrong thing by him (baby).*

Compared to their more accomplished sisters, dream-come-true mothers commenced maternity leave significantly earlier than other groups, usually approximately 5-6 weeks prior to their due dates. One member of this group was unemployed at the time of pregnancy and another had ceased work before 20 weeks. Most young-achievers were financially reliant on income and worked late into pregnancy. Two took accrued paid leave rather than unpaid maternity leave.

Working mothers within the literature

As we have seen in chapter 2, discourses of working mothers currently endorse two contradictory elements. On the one hand, there is an expectation that women will work and contribute in the public sphere (Filene, 1998). To do otherwise is considered a lesser choice (Filene, 1998). On the other hand there is an underlying assumption that mothers cannot be relied upon to concentrate on work or to contribute in the same way as other workers (Dally, 1982; Hattery, 2001; Kaplan, 1992) and criticism of mothers in terms of sick leave taken to care for children is common[18]. This understanding of mothers as less capable employees has resulted in a trend towards 'mommy tracking' or sidetracking mothers into less demanding jobs, ostensibly to accommodate their changed circumstances but also diminishing their chances of career advancement and promotion (Granrose & Kaplan, 1996; Hays, 1996; Thurer, 1994). Indeed, most career structures are, according to Hewlett (2002b), not especially accommodating of childbearing time out. Hewlett further suggests that older maternal age may represent the first opportunity for women to consider interrupting their careers (Hewlett, 2002c).

In this contested climate, it is little surprise that study participants describe a reluctance to announce pregnancies early, lest they be viewed less seriously than other workers.

Contemporary mother discourses also suggest that the infant needs almost exclusive maternal care (Forna, 1998; Glenn, 1994; Hays, 1996; Sheridan et al., 2002; Thurer, 1994) and commonly endorse a certain degree of criticism of 'selfish' mothers who put their careers before their children. There is a concomitant understanding of new mothering as incompatible with highly demanding professional lives (Kaplan, 1992). A telling example presents in Bettina Arndt's feature "Do political mums really know best?" (Age newspaper, 10/09/'02). In this article, Arndt questions a pregnant woman's choice to become a member of parliament and suggests that the woman is ill-advised and doing herself, her baby and her electorate a disservice[19] in pursuing her ambition.

Thus, it is scarcely surprising that older professional mothers might feel under pressure to fulfil work and mothering obligations and many study participants here describe feeling torn between their various obligations. Some employed extravagant measures to ensure that they fulfilled or more than fulfilled their work responsibilities lest they left themselves open to criticism. These measures included completion of major tasks prior to leaving and late commencement of maternity leave. As one mother succinctly described, 'I don't want them thinking I'm woolly brained just because I'm pregnant'.

What remains unclear in this study is why older mothers seem to have greater concerns around employment compared to younger professional women. One possible explanation may relate to the fact that many older mothers may have been 'tall poppies' in their field and thus may have had to compete in predominantly male arenas. Younger mothers, in contrast, may have been part of a more egalitarian work culture. This work versus mothering debate, particularly as it relates to older maternal age, is

---

[18] Why I don't like working with mothers. (2001, Dec). *SHE,* 43-44.
[19] Arndt, B. (10/09/2002). Do political mums really know best? The Age. Melbourne.

expanded in chapter 7. What follows now is a discussion of concerns voiced by study participants. At this stage, concerns related principally to pregnancy / fetal vulnerability and normality.

Concerns

In this study, perceptions of heightened vulnerability in the fetus were commonly expressed, particularly among the career women, but also among a substantial percentage of the dream-come-true mothers. This tendency was most marked among the women whose pregnancies were the result of prolonged efforts to conceive and many felt concerned lest they jeopardise the pregnancy in any way. This perception of increased vulnerability persisted despite little or no substantiating medical evidence.

Perceived vulnerability

As described in chapter 3, all participants here were considered to be carrying medically uncomplicated pregnancies and all were ultimately delivered of healthy term infants. Nonetheless, maternal impressions of 'last chance' or miracle pregnancies resulted in considerable self-imposed pressure to 'get it right'. Sally [career woman], for example, felt that this was her last chance to become a mother and, like Elizabeth in chapter 2, concentrated on doing it properly:

> *I thought this is my only chance and therefore that was a certain amount of pressure I was putting on myself, I guess ... every stage was just a day at a time, but it was not even the survival factor. My obstetrician had said it was possible that if they come too premature they could have neurological impairment as regards eyesight and hearing...*

Jane's [career woman] pregnancy was so anxiety-filled that she concentrated only on getting from one scan to the next. She explains:

> *And then when, when I was pregnant and they found twins and I lost that, lost one of the twins and I thought 'this is going to happen again, I'm going to lose the other one! I went through this sort of ... being healthy, waiting for the next scan, praying he's all right ...*

There was a sense of not wanting to tempt fate and this manifested as a reluctance to make too many plans, just in case. Many such women were happier for the doctor to make major decisions, rather than insist on informed or collaborative decision-making. Kristen [career woman] is a case in point and was unwilling to take on the responsibility of deciding whether or not to induce her pregnancy, because of worries about getting 'it wrong'. Here, she explains her attitude:

I had quite a few ultrasounds coming up to her birth, he [doctor] was just a little bit worried about the amount of fluid ... on the day she was born, I rang up and said I feel terrible and he said he could induce her, but the way he said it, he'd been worrying all along that she'd been going to be little, so the way he said, he sort of said it like 'I don't really want to do it'... and he wanted me to make a decision ... [I] was thinking I don't want to do anything wrong by her ... So I couldn't make the decision, so I said I'll do what you want me to do...

This notion of heightened vulnerability, mentioned briefly in the introduction and further developed in chapter 5, is supported within the literature. British psychologists, Berryman and Windridge (1995), who conducted the Leicester motherhood project, an extensive study of older [over 35] versus younger mothers, found that older mothers, in general, considered their babies to be at increased risk of damage or dying during pregnancy and delivery than did younger mothers. They additionally suggest that this perception of increased vulnerability relates to higher rates of medical surveillance in pregnancy in this group (Berryman & Windridge, 1995, p37).

Summary

In conclusion, the 'project' represents the first stage of transition to motherhood for the participants of this study, particularly career women. This approach to motherhood, employed particularly by mothers with significant career investment, involves a clearly defined trajectory of information gathering, preparation, planning and setting up the plan. Concerns around having the baby 'fit' into the parent's pre-existing lives, rather than changing to accommodate an infant, dominate pre-natal parental discussions. In contrast, dream-come-true mothers were less likely to be concerned about the baby 'fitting in' and in general adopted a 'going with the flow' attitude, accepting that 'things would change'. Young-achievers, although similar in some regards to career women, tended to be more accepting of, and adaptable to, life changes around the infant.

This unique approach of 'the project' sheds important light on the experiences of older primiparae. Close attention to the 'project' may promote greater understanding of the mothering experiences and concerns of this group of mothers and may thus inform future nursing strategies to assist transition among these women.

Although elaborate birth plans are often associated with older primiparae, the converse was found to be the case in this study. Participants here were concerned primarily with 'not jeopardising' the perceivably vulnerable pregnancy. Finally, for many participants, considerable tension around work-related decisions in the later stages of pregnancy is evident. This manifests in the late commencement of maternity leave, completion of major projects prior to leaving and the recruitment of replacements, personally supervised by the participants. An emphasis on not wasting time on maternity leave is also common. In general, the project is completed with the birth of a healthy baby, leaving the new mother ill equipped for the early days of mothering, which is addressed in the next chapter.

In chapter 5, early maternal experience as described by the study participants is discussed. Principal themes relate to the 'nightmare' of early mothering, succeeded by a stage of ambivalence and struggle.

CHAPTER 5
THE NIGHTMARE BEGINS

All the yelling and the carrying on, you've got to be joking! Like, what is wrong with you? Being older, I'm not interested in tha, ... 39 years doing your own thing, boy o boy! ... If you're a very reasonable or fairly practical sort of person "what the hell is wrong with you? ... Give me a break! I just can't work it out!

In the temporally ordered sequence of transition to motherhood, described in this study, 0-4 months were characterised to varying degrees, by feelings of helplessness and inadequacy among participants. Mothers described feeling 'overwhelmed' and 'drained' as they struggled with the responsibilities, fatigue and uncertainty of new motherhood. Although this stage of new mothering presents challenges for all women, the experiences of primiparae over 35 seem especially poignant and, in this study, women with significant career investment appeared to have exaggerated adjustment issues. Despite, or perhaps because of, elaborate prenatal preparation, these women often felt ill equipped for the early days of mothering and, for many, prenatal preparation had focused primarily on the production of the infant, rather than postpartum care.

Additionally, similar to older primigravidae in the literature, participants here frequently came to maternity with limited prior exposure to infants and fewer family or social supports. Despite extensive reading, many displayed a limited understanding of normal neonatal behaviour and concerns in the early days of mothering tended to encourage additional information searches. The resulting 'information overload' then left the inexperienced mother unable to decipher various suggestions for infant care. This surfeit of information without knowledge and perceptions of increased pregnancy vulnerability in turn contributed to feelings of anxiety in the new mother.

For their part, midwives and M&CHNs in the current study, identified the older primigravida's extensive prenatal preparation and reading as problematic and as contributing to the quandary of new mothering for this group. Central to the conundrum is the widely held belief that the requirements of appropriate childcare are self-evident and instinctively known. Age and prior experience also contributed to feelings among the mothers that they 'should know', resulting in reluctance to seek early assistance. Prenatal plans to 'avoid bad habits' and to prevent manipulation by the infant which guided the new mothers actions initially, also contributed to their difficulties.

In this chapter then, the 'nightmare' of early parenting is explored together with the struggles and ambivalence encountered by many of the study mothers. Stories are divided into two temporal periods, early mothering 1-4 weeks and mothering from 1-4 months. There is expectedly some overlap of experience though there are significant markers at these junctures. A clear trajectory of worry and uncertainty presented in the early days of mothering and was succeeded by struggle and ambivalence as women grappled with preserving something of their prior life, accommodating infant care and maintaining some personal space.

The transition to motherhood / early mothering 1-4 weeks

"During the early weeks of motherhood at home, the new mother is plunged into a state of inner disequilibrium and external upheaval quite unlike any encountered in adult life. Still 'wide open' from her expansive physical and emotional experiences of pregnancy and giving birth, she also suffers from frequent rude awakenings ... and insufficient sleep. Tiredness, hormonal fluctuations, drastic bodily changes ... and painful stitches, all add to the emotional turmoil evoked by contagious exposure to the primitive needs of the baby."

(Raphael-Leff, 1991, pp. 354-355)

New motherhood is characterised by adaptive changes and challenges for all mothers and the early months following birth are commonly regarded as particularly challenging (Antonucci & Mikus, 1988; Barclay & Lloyd, 1996; Cappuccini & Cochrane, 2000; Cowan & Cowan, 1995; Leifer, 1980; Nelson, 2003b; Pridham & Chang, 1992). Becoming a mother is recognised as a life change of such magnitude (Rogan et al., 1997), as to rival that of marriage (Leifer, 1980; Lopata, 1971; Rossi, 1968). The first month postpartum is marked by maternal fatigue, frustration, concerns about the infant and about the ability to mother. This stage is frequently considered to be the most difficult period during the transition to motherhood (Rogan et al., 1997; Rubin, 1984). Feeling 'unready' for the changes associated with new maternity also features prominently among the accounts of new mothers, regardless of age (Barclay et al., 1997; McVeigh, 1997b). Transition occurs as mothers address difficulties and meet challenges (Chick & Meleis, 1986; Pridham & Chang, 1992) and continues until caring for the infant "no longer seems unfamiliar or unpredictable" (Pridham & Chang, 1992, p. 205). Although new motherhood, as a time of major change and upheaval for all mothers, is well documented, the anxieties and struggles of the participants of this study seem unusually poignant. The older mother often enters maternity having prepared elaborately but, nonetheless, may be ill equipped for the early days of mothering. Prenatal preparation, for the participants of this study, focused largely on the production of a healthy infant and, as discussed in the preceding chapter, the 'project' was completed with the birth of a healthy infant, which then gave rise to worries and concerns not anticipated by the mothers. In general, early mothering (1-4 weeks) for study participants was characterised by feelings of helplessness and exhaustion, information overload and a mismatch between preparation and subsequent experience. Terrifying anxieties and a tendency towards vigilance are also noted.

The project is completed

Many of the women in this study expressed feeling that once the infant was born healthy, everything else would be manageable. Harriet [career woman] explains:

I concentrated only on it being healthy, everything else could be dealt with later. If I couldn't breastfeed it or it cried at night, well, we could deal with that, once it was normal...

The feeling that 'nature would kick in' was commonly expressed and is in keeping with contemporary mothering discourses. Socially, there is a widely held belief that the requirements of appropriate childcare are instinctively known (Hays, 1996) and during pregnancy the participants of this study mostly expected that 'things would fall into place' once the baby was born.

Jane [career woman] explains:

I expected that once I had the baby I would just be a natural mother and it would be easy...

That is not to say that the women were unconcerned about mothering. Indeed, several women described wondering pre-natally how they might 'cope' with an infant. However, immediate concerns about the perceivably vulnerable pregnancy precluded any real reflection on the next stage. The busyness of the women's pre-maternity lives and late commencement of maternity leave also left little time for thought. Contingency plans for some participants included an early return to work if 'being at home proved too difficult'.

Following birth and immediate postpartum euphoria, the new mother was confronted with the myriad concerns of her new role. For the women of this study, there was a clearly recognisable void after the 'project' ended and many described feeling really lost and helpless. Difficulties included feeling

97

overwhelmed with information, suffering fatigue and feeling that the expected support in hospital did not eventuate. Some participants seemed to suffer a paralysing degree of helplessness in the hours following birth and describe an inability to make decisions about their own care whilst in hospital, to the extent that they would seek permission to get out of bed or to go to the toilet.

Feeling helpless

Although many women of all ages feel uncertain and out of their depth after a first birth, the experiences of the older participants of this study, especially career women, seem exaggerated. Kelly [career woman] explains:

I had no idea what to do!

Jane [career woman] was so mesmerised by her experience that she was uncertain following delivery if she was allowed to get up:

I was not sure if I was allowed to get up, so I rang for the nurse

This level of helplessness is seldom seen among younger women, but in this study was common to older mothers irrespective of career investment. For many, being alone with the baby was a very frightening experience, particularly for those women who had had limited prior exposure to children. Jennifer [dream-come-true] expresses her concerns:

Is she going to choke? Have I put her down properly? You know you have her by the side of the bed, is she going to survive the night, sort of thing? You're thinking to yourself, if only ... I'd burst into tears ... I felt that you were left very much to your own devices, there was not a great deal of support there with some of the people [midwives] ... I rang and said 'could you please just, just take her for 5 minutes so I could have a shower ... And she said, no no no, you need to settle her and this, that and the other! And I sat there and I just lost it ... even with my husband there I felt helpless ...

98

Information overload / mismatch

As described in chapter 4, there is a clearly demonstrated tendency among older, well-educated mothers to read and to gather extensive information in preparation for motherhood and, in this study, participants' prenatal reading had centred largely on areas of anticipated concern such as breastfeeding and sleep difficulties in infants. However, despite extensive reading, mothers display a limited understanding of normal neonatal behaviour and a seeming inability to distinguish normal behaviour from more significant concerns. Compounding the difficulties for this group of women was limited prior exposure to infants and limited family or social support. Mothers were often unable to decipher the manifold suggestions for infant care uncovered during reading and did not have a reference framework to make sense of the recruited information. This in turn led to further information searches and confusion, resulting in what one mother describes as an 'information overload'. As in the preceding chapter, this trend was most commonly seen among career women and to a lesser extent, young-achievers. Anita [young-achiever] explains:

You're just inundated with lots and lots of information, I'm sick of reading,

They prepare themselves the way they think they should

For the midwives and M&CHNs, the older primigravida's extensive prenatal preparation and reading was frequently viewed as problematic, inappropriate and as contributing to the difficulties of new mothering for women over 35. A mismatch between the information gathered and that required is identified by Lucy and Maria (midwives):

They actually tend to prepare themselves the way they think they should be prepared ... they may not have prepared themselves the way we think they should've prepared...
Lucy

The ones ... reading a lot about motherhood ... and how the baby will sleep are really focused ... books regarding motherhood and pregnancy and all that ... things don't always go according to the books ... they come in with these set ideas about how things are going to go, it doesn't always go like that...
Maria

The tendency on the part of the women to solicit multiple opinions was also poorly regarded by the midwives, as Joan [midwife] explains:

They tend to want to know 'what do you think? And then 'you too' oh, and you too ... and then it's conflicting advice! ... Rather than take a little bit of what everyone says, listening to what everyone says and you'll be right as rain, but it's got to be right, is what she said right? And what she said was right too?

In general, there was a poor fit between information gathered and that required in the early days of parenting. This mismatch contributed to maternal anxiety and many mothers described feeling totally unprepared for looking after an infant.

Totally unprepared

Inappropriate preparation and overwhelming responsibility epitomised the immediate postpartum experience for many participants, again mostly career women. These women described feeling 'shocked' and 'out of control' as the requirements of parenting became evident. Fatigue and pain compounded their experience. Gayle [career woman] explains:

I don't think there is anyone who can tell you the magnitude of the task, you can read whatever you like, but until you are actually in it, embroiled in it, it's the weirdest thing, that you cannot have any understanding of it at all, until you're the character in the role...

This feeling of being unprepared for new motherhood is commonly found in the literature and affects all age groups. Barclay et al. (1997) describe a category of 'unready' as a fundamental concept during the transition to motherhood. McVeigh (1997b), in her study of early mothering (0-6 weeks) experiences of 100 first-time mothers in Sydney, found similarly that the participants described 'feeling unprepared' for early mothering. In addition, a considerable number of researchers have concluded that current educational strategies available to pregnant women provide insufficient preparation (Cooke, 2000; Emmanuel et al., 2001; Mahoney, 2000; Nolan, 1997). Although feeling 'unprepared' is frequently associated with new motherhood, a noted difference in this study is the depth of anxiety the participants, particularly career women, suffer in association with feeling unprepared. A tendency to berate themselves for not being prepared also presents and is considered in a later section of this chapter. Going home from hospital marked a major event in the lives of the new mothers and, for the majority of career women, a time of great distress.

Going home

This juncture was characterised by a lack of time, fatigue and pressure to 'get everything done'. Breastfeeding difficulties and erratic infant schedules contributed to feelings of spiralling 'out of control'. Laura [career woman] explains:

It was just a nightmare, like seriously a nightmare for 2 months ... I was tired all the time and I just seemed to be waking, feeding, waking, feeding and I felt just awful! I was tired all the time, so I was not really enjoying it that much and I found being home really, really difficult ... she had her good days and her bad days and her bad days could've been just not settling all day and crying and not wanting to be put down, you pretty much couldn't do anything ... even though the day just seemed to go and I'd look back and think I didn't get a chance to do anything other than eat or clean ...

Similar to Rubin's findings, many of the women in this study tried to replicate the exact conditions familiar to them from the hospital. Rubin (1984) found that the new mother "will bathe her baby with the same kind of soap and in the same procedure and dress the baby with the same kind and amount of clothing as 'they' did in the hospital" (p. 40). This imitation of the 'expert model', according to Rubin, was likely to provide a "probabilistic certainty in a stage of great uncertainty" (p. 40). In this study, women with little prior experience of children were particularly likely to replicate hospital models and once again the career women are highly represented. In their study of postpartum adjustment in first-time mothers, Fleming, Flett, Ruble and Shaul (1988) found similarly that maternal adequacy was closely linked to prior experience with children. Here Rosie [career woman] explains her approach:

What we had at the hospital didn't transfer here, like my friend had given me some supplies and methods and they didn't work ... and the ones [nappies] they had at the hospital didn't transfer, didn't have the same material and the same services. You didn't know where anything was, even though I'd tried to organise it, it just wasn't[the same] ...

Dream-come-true mothers, although also nervous and unsure, did not appear to suffer the same degree of unease, as Janet explains:

> *As hard as it is, it's better when you go home, you don't have to worry about people coming in the room [in hospital] all the time ... you had different midwives everyday ... I was fed up because every shift [there] was a different midwife, who told me something different ...*

In this study, there was a tendency among the career women and young-achievers particularly, to require clear specific guidelines in the early days of mothering and the absence of clear guidelines made this stage very uncertain.

Wanting clear specific guidelines

Many women spoke of 'just wanting an answer' and this tendency was described succinctly by one maternal and child health nurse as a 'recipe for bringing up baby'. Sorting through the various information and suggestions proved difficult, with much of the offered advice appearing to contradict earlier suggestions. Harriet [career woman] explains:

> *The worse part was though, even in the hospital, there were conflicting stories on, about how much he should be drinking and [if] you should burp him, that sort of thing!*

Anita [young-achiever]:

> *When the midwife came I said to her 'how long should I be breastfeeding for? And she said it just depends on the baby, so I was sitting there an hour and a half and an hour after that... I asked my doctor next day and he said half an hour is fine, you're taking too long, I just wanted an answer...*

A lack of specificity and clarity of the maternal role is identified in the literature as contributing to maternal angst for all mothers. Mercer (1986), found that a lack of clear role descriptions made the early days of mothering very difficult for many mothers and lack of role consensus is frequently identified as contributing to transition difficulty, in a variety of circumstances (Burr, Leigh, Day &

Constandine, 1979; Chick & Meleis, 1986; Mercer, 1986). In addition to feeling unprepared, many women here described a sense of unreality in the early days of mothering, described below.

Sense of unreality

In this study, several mothers spoke of expecting the baby to disappear or of being surprised at the baby's 'real' appearance and this tendency is displayed almost exclusively by career women. Here Jane [career woman] seems amazed at her baby's humanity:

He had all this hair and he looked so perfect and I thought, the first thing that came to my mind was ' how did he come out of me? I would see babies and funnily enough, I'd see them and I could not imagine my baby looking like that it was like em, just wasn't real, I couldn't picture it ...

Karine too [dream-come-true, IVF twins] felt very removed from her experience:

It's funny, I still look at these and I can't believe I had a big belly on me! That they're actually from me ... I still can step outside that experience and be bowled over by it ...

This concept of 'unreality' is difficult to locate within the literature and of the sources obtained the notion is more usually expressed pre-natally, for example, Schmied and Lupton (2001). Schmied and Lupton explore body images and impressions of pregnancy and report a sense of unreality among the expectant mothers' accounts and Mercer (1986) reports a sense of wonderment in the accounts of mothers immediately following birth. Here, the sense of unreality seemed to relate to maternal reluctance to engage emotionally in the pregnancy and, in this study, the tendency manifested principally among those mothers with 'last chance' pregnancies. A co-existent level of anxiety is described by many of the study's older mothers.

Terrifying anxieties

Terrifying anxieties troubled many participants, despite the associated neonates all being healthy term infants. Maternal perceptions of heightened infant vulnerability were common and, in general, were not supported by medical evidence. As before, this tendency presents more commonly among the career women accounts. Indeed, several women felt their worries were 'obsessive', but nonetheless felt powerless to control them. Abigail [career woman] explains:

103

I worry about her getting sick or dying! All the time, so much so I sometimes think it's too obsessive!

Keeping busy

Many of the participants kept their pre-natal worries under check by keeping busy. Whilst this was a feature of their busy working lives, for some this was also a conscious effort and helped prevent negative thoughts from intruding. Jennifer [dream-come-true] explains:

Mostly, I kept myself very busy so that I wouldn't worry, I kept myself occupied, I did not let myself think, ... the responsibility, whether she'd be normal or not, all those things, all these worries...

A resultant lack of engagement and distancing from the pregnancy was noted and, as discussed in chapter 4, was most marked among the more professional women. Although distancing strategies were quite successful at keeping major concerns at bay during pregnancy, birth tended to trigger a cascade of emotions and unresolved feelings. Abigail [career woman] explains:

I couldn't give my 100% attention to the baby, with my thoughts and that, because I was thinking about other things as well and that made me feel very helpless...

Still others had scarcely addressed the possibility of having a live and healthy infant and, for these women, impending birth proved a considerable source of anxiety. Such was Jane's [career woman] anxiety around birth that she feared she would die during caesarean section:

I was very nervous on the day, because the doctor had talked to me about blood clots and all sorts of things like that, so I sort of ... I was sort of lying there thinking 'Oh my God' I wanted to be able to live to see my baby and em, I even thought about my will and everything...

Anxieties around normality and perceived infant vulnerability were more pronounced among the career women and although dream-come-true mothers also worried extravagantly, their fears seemed to encompass a less expansive range. This finding may relate in part to the career women's exposure to a myriad of possible complications uncovered during extensive reading. Additional surveillance, such as ultrasonic scans and genetic testing, may have also exacerbated concerns. For all women, the level of anxiety seemed to relate to the length of time it had taken to achieve pregnancy, with the women who had conceived quickly worrying least. In particular, women availing of IVF technology were exposed to additional risks and complications and became intimately familiar with age-related poorer conception rates. It follows that impressions of 'last chance / miracle' pregnancy might imbue the process of childbearing with heightened significance for these women. Such women may then feel under intense pressure to 'get it right', as indeed may health professionals involved in their care. Holt (1988) understood this notion well, describing the trend towards later childbearing and lower birth rates as "aggravating the pressure on parents and obstetricians alike to make every baby a perfect baby" (p. 172). Additionally, many mothers benefiting from IVF technologies bring anxieties and unresolved issues to their transition to motherhood (Imeson & McMurray, 1996; Sandelowski, 1995a) that may also contribute to later perceptions of infant vulnerability.

Infant vulnerability

In this study, impressions of infant vulnerability presented more frequently among the accounts of the older mothers, irrespective of level of education. This notion of greater fetal / infant risk is also found within the scant literature addressing the experiences of mothers over 35. For example, Berryman and Windridge (1995) and Windridge and Berryman (1999) found that older mothers in general considered their babies to be at greater risk of damage or dying during pregnancy and delivery than younger mothers. Views of the pregnancy as 'last chance' seemed to contribute to this impression of vulnerability among participants here and, although this notion was difficult to locate in the literature, some parallels were found. For example, Payne (2002) conducted an analysis of the term 'elderly primigravida' for her doctoral thesis and discussed "motherhood as a limited opportunity" (p. 135). She found that her study participants [over 35 years] frequently regarded pregnancy as an exceptional achievement, which resulted in heightened concerns about the pregnancy / baby.

In this study, impressions of fetal risk were not necessarily related to medical complication and are perhaps explained by Ford and Hodnett's findings of subjective risk appraisal. Ford and Hodnett (1990), whose study centred on women hospitalised during pregnancy and does not specifically refer to older mothers, discovered that pregnant women's appraisal of risk was subjective and related to perceived threat to the fetus. This understanding of risk was found to be "independent of and sometimes divergent from, the risk status determined by medical personnel" (p. 47). Similarly, levels of maternal anxiety in this study appeared to relate more to perceived risk than to actual medical complication and may in part relate to being deemed 'at risk'.

'At risk'

Here, many participants described their pre-pregnancy health as above average, which is consistent with findings discussed in the introductory chapter (Berryman et al., 1999; Ventura, 1989). However, on interacting with the health system, the older mother often learnt that, despite her pre-pregnancy health, she was regarded as being 'at risk' related to age alone. There is some suggestion within the literature that this labelling of 'elderly primigravida' as 'high risk' contributes to a perception of heightened fetal vulnerability (Berryman et al., 1999, Payne, 2002). For Della, [M&CHN], this labelling had a major impact on maternal competency:

> *They write down elderly primip. It gets written in hospital, ... it comes on the mothers' summaries ... and the mothers will point it out to you 'I'm an elderly primip' ... they're made to feel more vulnerable ... like you're a special case!*

A poignant example also presents in Payne's (2002) thesis. Payne describes during interview, how she, as a fit and healthy primigravida aged over 35, had planned to have a home birth, but after visiting her doctor and absorbing a very negative medical view of age associated risk, she began to see herself as 'at risk' (Giddings & Wood, 2002).

In this study, impressions of infant vulnerability also gave rise to a tendency towards vigilance.

Vigilance

This tendency towards vigilance was demonstrated by several of the study's older mothers, again principally, though not exclusively, career women. Many describe being afraid to shower even whilst the baby slept, in case the baby would have some difficulty and the mother might be unavailable. Others reported waking with a start and worrying that something might have happened to the infant whilst the mother was 'off guard'. Several described having their only occasions of deep sleep when their partner was home and caring for the baby. Then, they felt they could relax and relinquish the care and vigilance to him. Interestingly, this trend towards vigilance is not described in any of the studies accessed, such as Barclay et al. (1997); Feldman and Nash (1986); Gottesman (1992); Leifer (1980);

McVeigh (1997a); Mercer (1986) and Rubin (1984). However, parallels are found in studies of transition to motherhood for mothers of premature infants cared for in special care / intensive care facilities, such as, Doering, Moser and Dracup (2000) and Hurst (2001). Angela's [dream-come-true] example of not sleeping except over her infant's cot is perhaps an extreme example:

In the beginning I was hanging over the cot, afraid to go to sleep, in case something would happen ... because you're at home, constantly looking after her day and night, you have this constant fear that if something happens to her you're going to be the one that's at fault, you're going to be the one to blame, so you're constantly checking, I remember checking on her 100 times when she was sleeping ...

This period of vigilance of the baby was somewhat muted by about four weeks of age and some mothers describe falling into an exhausted sleep one night and upon wakening several hours later realised that the infant had survived this lapse in attention. This understanding in turn increased the mother's confidence in sleeping on subsequent nights. Together with the helplessness and anxiety of the early days of mothering, participants here spoke of feeling that others presumed they would know a certain amount about caring for an infant, and for these women, a reluctance to seek help initially was common.

People presume you would know

Age and prior experience contributed to this feeling among the mothers that they 'should know' and several participants spoke of perceiving health professionals to be dismissive of their concerns. Rachel [career woman] explains:

I think there's an expectation and a lot of the nursing staff, ... because you're older, [think] that you instinctively know what to do, but I don't think you do ... it makes you sometimes feel a little bit, not inferior but ... because you don't know what to do ... so the hardest part for me was after I had Bradley ... I had that expectation of myself, just a few looks or comments or whatever, you think should I have known that? Was that a dumb sort of question, do you think? Does that mean that question was a dumb question?

107

Focus group midwives and M&CHNs showed a clear understanding of the women's reluctance to ask questions, but dealt with it in different ways [Appendix C]. Some, like Dorothy [midwife] tended to cue into the woman's needs and to offer assistance before the woman broached the subject, effectively giving her permission to seek help:

They're not sure whether to ask for help or not, they're sure they should know and they're usually so relieved when you offer it...

Whereas Cathy [M&CHN] felt the women's fear of 'losing face' contributed to their difficulties:
A lot of them hang off, because they believe they should know it and they like, they try everything they know and then they're in dire straits...

There was a general understanding of the women's psychological vulnerability, despite their outward show of confidence. Although most women in this study expressed multiple concerns in the first months of parenting, a particular emergent pattern prompted enquiry about specifics and women were subsequently asked about the 'hardest thing to accommodate in the early days'. Four areas of major concern were identified by participants.

Major concerns
The principal areas of concern described by the mothers are ordered here by level of reporting: lack of sleep / extreme fatigue; concerns about the baby / breastfeeding difficulties; concerns about mothering and finally, lack of support / feeling isolated at home. These areas of concern were common to all older mothers in the study, irrespective of social standing and educational / employment status, though again there was a tendency towards exaggerated concern among those mothers who had read and prepared extensively.

Lack of sleep / maternal exhaustion
In this study, all participants expressed concerns about fatigue and lack of sleep, though again, exhaustion was more pronounced among the older mothers. The depth of fatigue seemed to vary little between 'career women' and 'dream-come-true' mothers, with many women feeling their functional capacity was affected by extreme fatigue. The words 'dangerous', 'terrible' and 'unstuck', feature in their accounts, as Cassie [career woman] explains:

*And again going back to sleep deprivation, that's when things become unstuck, I think ...
and you fight with each other and the clients get on your nerves...*

Gayle [career woman] discovered a newfound respect for sleep-deprived individuals:

*I now have a new respect for people who do terrible things out of sleep deprivation ... I
used to think, how could you do that to your child and I actually think it's possible now ...
one person was telling me that they were bathing their child and the next minute they
realised that he was under the water and they'd gone to sleep with their eyes open...*

Women from the young-achievers group also reported feeling both tired and very tired and made
serious efforts to address the lack of sleep. Overall, though, they seemed to be less seriously affected by
fatigue and more accepting that fatigue was part and parcel of mothering. Kim [young-achiever]
explains:

*I knew I'd lose sleep ... I was saying at work before I left 'oh my baby's not going to cry,
it's going to sleep 8 hours at night ... they just laughed and said 'you're being really
realistic then!'*

Age-related fatigue

At this stage fatigue was frequently identified by the participants as associated with the aging body and
this theme is discussed in greater detail in chapter 7. The midwives also identified an increase of
fatigue among the older women and felt exhaustion was compounded by the fact that the women were
less likely to rest or nap while the baby slept. They also raised the suggestion that extreme fatigue in
the older mother might have physiological antecedents.

*They've got less patience, as you get older, you find you're tireder, your body doesn't
bounce back like it does in your twenties! So they do find it harder...*
Jill [midwife]

109

They are so tired, suffering from exhaustion ... [though] it's not just related to tiredness,
they just don't know how to look after themselves, they don't know how to put themselves to
bed ... they don't understand that 10 minutes sleep might revive them...
Lucy [midwife]

Age-related fatigue within the literature

Overall, there is a common understanding of fatigue in the early days of mothering for all mothers
(Barclay et al., 1997; Crouch & Manderson, 1993; McVeigh, 1997a, 1997b) irrespective of age or
parity. There is additionally no clear consensus on age-related extreme fatigue within the literature,
though the weight of opinion seems to suggest that degrees of maternal fatigue do not relate
particularly to maternal age. MacArthur, Lewis & Knox (1991) conducted a large scale (n = 11,701)
follow-up study of women delivering at the Birmingham Maternity hospital [England] between the
years 1978-85. They found that extreme maternal fatigue was reported with a higher frequency among
older mothers, particularly primiparae from higher social classes. Mercer (1986), in her study of 294
primiparous women, also found an age-related increase in reported fatigue among older participants
and Rubin (1984), discussed pervasive postpartum fatigue related to anaemia and birth exhaustion, but
made no mention of age-related extremes.

Overall, the evidence seems to favour the converse argument. Australians Brown et al. (1994)
conducted a survey of women giving birth in Victoria in a two-week period in 1993 (n = 1331) and
observed that tiredness was a pervasive problem affecting all groups of women, unrelated to age or
parity. Glazener et al. (1995) also found that maternal fatigue was unrelated to parity of delivery mode
(n = 1391). Green and Kafetsios (1997), in their study of women aged 21-35 years (n = 1285) found
that at 6 weeks postpartum, tiredness was the most important variable in regard to postpartum
experience, though no age-related differences were mentioned. Americans Pugh and Milligan (1993),
discussed hormonal and physiological changes as likely predictors of maternal fatigue and Berryman et
al. (1999) disputed commonly held views of age-related fatigue, suggesting it more likely related to
higher numbers of breastfeeding mothers in this group.

In this study, maternal fatigue was pervasive and common to all older mothers. It may be that there is
some physiological basis for this premise, or it may simply relate to high levels of breastfeeding effort,
pre-natal anxiety, late commencement of maternity leave and poorer postpartum support. Many of the
participants mentioned pre-natal fatigue, particularly towards the end of pregnancy, which perhaps
added to the depth of postpartum fatigue experienced. Following fatigue and sleep concerns, most

110

frequently cited worries included concerns about the infant and about the quality of mothering. Those concerns are now explored.

Concerns about the baby / concerns about mothering

These dual concerns dominated the experiences of all the study mothers and are dealt with together as they are so closely linked. The trend was for older mothers, irrespective of educational / employment status, to express a greater level of concern than did the younger mothers. Feelings of uncertainty and incompetence were commonly expressed, particularly worries about doing the right thing and 'not knowing what to do'. Here

Laura, [career woman] expresses sentiments commonly associated with career women:

> *What am I doing wrong, I'm stressed out, like why is she crying now? I've just given her a feed and changed her nappy ... You try to work things out, ... Am I doing the right thing? ... Hopefully nothing happens to her, hopefully she's not sick!*

For Angela [dream-come-true] terrors related to infant demise drove her to her GP several times a week, abating only after approximately 4 months of age:

> *And when she was 3-4 months old I can remember going to the doctors 4 times a week and my doctor used to say 'blimey! You've got bags under your eyes! Go home and get some sleep.'*

All mothers in the study, irrespective of age, education or accomplishment, were concerned about their mothering abilities in the early days of parenting. This was similar to Mercer's (1986) finding that the "level of interest in and concern about mothering" was similarly distributed among all age groups, at one-month postpartum (p. 129). However, the intensity of worry among older mothers in this study seems particularly striking.

What if I get it wrong?

Worries about reading the situation 'wrong' and feelings of overwhelming dependency compounded the frightening experience, particularly for those women with limited social support. In this study, this tendency was equally demonstrated among all older mothers. Petra [career woman] explains:

111

When you don't know if you're doing the right thing, that was, I think that was the most
frustrating ... [you're] used to, you know, I'll do this path and ... and you're quite
confident that it ... Oh my God! What if something goes wrong? ... When someone's life is
depending on you!

Kelly [career woman] felt overwhelmed:

I think the feeling of total dependency on you, he relies on me for everything I can't
remember ever being so overwhelmed by anything!

Fears of inadvertently damaging the infant were also commonly voiced by both categories of older mothers and are clearly related to notions of maternal accountability, articulated in contemporary discourses (Thurer 1994). These notions of maternal responsibility for the child's emotional welfare, particularly in regard to avoiding psychological damage to the infant, have been present in discourses from the 1960s/1970s (Kaplan, 1992; Thurer, 1994). There is also the suggestion that mothers might damage the infant as much by omission as by commission. A poignant, if somewhat dated example presents in the advice Penelope Leach (1975) offers to the unfortunate mother of a *jumpy* baby:

"... caring for him can be even enjoyable if it is seen as a challenge. The challenge is simply whether every day can be got through without him ever being frightened or made to jump. It takes constant thought. It means never being distracted so that the overhead light is suddenly switched on in a dark room, never sitting down to feed him just where the telephone is going to ring in his face, never running downstairs with him under your arm to answer the door, never pulling his vest over his head because the strings are in a knot."

(Leach, 1975, p. 94)

As well as an emphasis on maternal accountability for her infant's 'normal' development, mother blaming for 'abnormal' development is common in discourses (Cooey, 1999; Thurer, 1994). For the women of this study, out of time with their peers and prey to social censure, this concern of avoiding psychological damage to the infant was often distressing. Jennifer [dream-come-true], for example, worried extravagantly that her daughter's refusal to have an afternoon nap might prove injurious:

Now if someone had to say to me look, she might have to miss a sleep, then I'd know! ... Oh
my God, this terrible fear and people instil it in you! Really! she should be asleep! and you
think 'oh my God!' what am I doing to my child? Am I going to harm her?

112

In addition to concerns about damaging the infant many participants, again principally career women, appeared to attach undue significance to the 'little things' such as burping the infant sufficiently or interpreting infant noises.

Worrying about the little things / disproportionate concerns

In this study, many women described feeling very unprepared for the everyday care of an infant and concerns such as positioning the baby for sleep and dressing the infant in the correct weight of clothing were troublesome. Although uncertainty and worry are generally considered to be part and parcel of new mothering (Barclay et al., 1997; McVeigh, 1997b; Mercer, 1986), the level of concern expressed by participants here seemed disproportionate. Compounding the anxiety was the exaggerated but very real concern of SIDS and mothers were terrified of over-heating the infant. So great was this fear of overheating the infant that, when I went to interview mothers in the depth of winter, I discovered that many mothers had closed heating vents in the infant's room and put the baby to bed in light clothing and with a single blanket. They would then worry when the infant was unsettled at night without considering the possibility that he/she might be cold. Many struggled to maintain perspective. Rachel [career woman] explains her concerns:

> *Our biggest concern with Bradley is that I don't know how to dress him, I'm frightened if he's too hot ... or under-dressing him ... you're frightened if you are doing the right thing or the wrong thing or whatever ... and being in bed, so I'd read up on SIDS and I knew how to make his cot up, that was my biggest concern and that still is!*

> *And even the other day, when I was driving, he had a long sleeved top on and I was actually a bit warm in the car, so I turned the cooler on and I'm thinking, 'Oh blow, should I have a breeze blowing round the car, which isn't a gale breeze now I think about it, but do I have that breath of fresh air around the car or is he going to get frostbite, what should I be doing?*

As we chatted in the kitchen after the interview, Rachel expressed her concerns about dressing her infant appropriately for the weather. She found it difficult to know 'exactly' how to interpret my suggestion that the infant required one layer more than she did, that extra layer usually being a wrap or blanket. It transpired that she would like me to write out a list of what constituted appropriate clothing for a newborn, in five-degree increments. Additionally, she required me to clearly explain whether a hat referred to a woollen or cotton hat and at what sort of temperature one would change from one to the other. When her infant needed socks was another concern.

This mind-numbing level of concern was such a surprise to me that I discussed it at length with a number of friends, colleagues and family, including my mother, herself a veteran mother of ten. Her response was to laughingly reply 'Thank God I didn't have to do parenting, as well as everything else', which made me think about what was so different about the experiences of contemporary women. I followed up on the concept in subsequent interviews and became aware of a tendency to regard caring for the infant as an 'awesome responsibility', which abated only when the mother started to think of her infant as a 'little person', at around 3-4 months, when the infant started to smile and respond to the mother. This concept of the 'little person' is explored in the following chapter. In addition to concerns around day-to-day care of the infant, breastfeeding proved considerably more challenging than anticipated for many participants.

Breastfeeding difficulties

Breastfeeding posed a major concern for many mothers, with poor supply a particular problem for the older women. Ten older mothers had ceased breastfeeding in the early weeks, many after a heroic battle with supply augmentation devices and dietary supplements. All cited insufficient supply as the reason for weaning the infant and some women were still struggling mentally with their experience, several months later. This finding of age-related poor supply is not well addressed in the literature, though popular wisdom among midwives and lactation consultants suggests that women who avail of fertility technologies frequently have their dreams of breastfeeding thwarted by insufficient supply. Within the literature, insufficient supply is thought to affect only "a very small number of women" (Monaghan, Braund & Brodribb, 2001, p. 1, see also Fallows, 1994; Howard, 1990; Kitzinger, 1987; Lawrence & Lawrence, 1999). Indeed, the World Health Organisation [WHO](1991) suggest that only 1-5% of women are physiologically incapable of sustaining lactation sufficient to feed an infant. Associated lactation difficulties are thought to be 'easily managed' or preventable by education and adequate maternal support (Monaghan et al., 2001; WHO, 2002). Although there is no denying the importance of breastfeeding support (Dennis, Hodnett, Gallop & Chalmers, 2002; Neifert, Seacat & Jobe, 1985), limited support alone fails to account for the rate of approximately 45% lactation insufficiency described by the older study participants and it would seem that participants' experiences did indeed relate to lactation insufficiency, as each of the mothers concerned described being approached by her

114

maternal and child health nurse as a result of infant weight loss or failure to thrive. Kelly [career woman] explains her experience:

I go to the welfare [M&CHN] and they say 'oh, he's very underweight! And I say 'is it serious, should I be worried about it'? So I end up worrying and then I was scared he was too thin and he was just breastfed, so they said to top him up.

For Annie, [dream-come-true] being unable to breastfeed was particularly distressing and she went to considerable lengths to 'bring her milk in':

I really wanted to feed but I can't do every 2 hours ... up until yesterday I was wanting to continue going and trying to get it in and whatever it took ... like Mum had to help me pump it out, ... it just took so long ... there's just nothing there, it's still soft, It's just being awful! [crying] ... there's just nothing there! My sister in law had her little boy two days later and she said her milk is squirting out, squirting him in the face.

Cited causes for insufficient supply include: pituitary malfunction (Lawrence & Lawrence, 1999); insufficient breast development (Neifert et al., 1985); breast surgery (Brodribb, 1992); pharmacological factors (Hale, 2000); and hormonal abnormalities (Brodribb, 1997), including polycystic ovarian syndrome (Marasco, Marmet & Shell, 2000). Interestingly, polycystic ovarian syndrome is frequently associated with IVF therapy (Monash IVF 2001) and of the ten older mothers unable to breast feed 5 were recipients of IVF / fertility treatments, although no conclusions can be drawn from this small study sample. For the mothers who continued to breastfeed, the journey was often no less arduous. Gayle [career woman] explains:

I had her on Thursday morning and by Saturday I was on an absolute treadmill, it was taking over my life, ... I think the feeding thing was the hardest...

However, for the four mothers who returned to full-time work prior to 6 months postpartum, continuing to breast feed and express milk for their infants in their absence somewhat assuaged their guilt. Gayle [career woman] explains:

And even in my mums' group of all the women who went back [to work] none of them are feeding, except for me ... and that sort of relieves my guilt ...

Finally, lack of support / feeling isolated at home presents as the fourth major concern for study mothers and is discussed as follows.

Lack of support / feeling isolated at home

Lack of family support, particularly parental support, was a major issue for many study participants and the experience was compounded for several women who had very elderly or frail parents. For two of the career women, poor relationships with their own mothers precluded all but the most minimal contact after birth. For another three women, their mothers had died some time earlier and a further three participants lived a significant distance from parents or family. Gayle [career woman] for example, had no close family or friends to whom she could entrust the care of her infant and her husband's long hours added to her burden:

Well the thing is ... we've got no family here, we have no one that I know, friend-wise, that have children of a similar age, I don't have any family support, I have a husband who works long hours and really, I can't ask him to do any more than he is doing and my mother is dead ... if she was still alive it would be different ... she was all for the family ...

As discussed briefly in the introductory chapter, later timing mothers often live some distance from family (Ambler Walter, 1986; Cook, 1993; Reece, 1995) and as early as 1967, Rubin suggested an association between older primiparity and limited support, describing such mothers as having "no women kinfolk other than a mother somewhere" (1967a, p. 344). Although contemporary trends of increasing maternal age make older primiparity less of a rarity, for the women of the current study it was sometimes a profoundly isolating experience and many mothers felt poorly supported. Lack of maternal support is generally considered to augur poorly for subsequent maternal adjustment. Indeed, maternal support is underscored in a host of studies as an important mediator of adjustment (Barclay et al., 1997; Fleming et al., 1988; Green & Kafetsios, 1997; Kramer, Chalmers, Hodnett, Sevkovskaya, Dzikovich, Shapiro. et al. 2001[PROBIT study group]; Reece, 1995; Tarkka, 2003; Tarkka & Paunonen, 1996) and it follows that a lack thereof may prove problematic. However, we shall see in chapter 6 that this is not necessarily the case for this study's participants. For mothers in this study, the

116

spouse / partner provided the bulk of support, although this was not always a satisfactory arrangement as many of the fathers worked very long hours. There was a tendency for childcare and decisions around the baby to fall largely to the mother, in what De Beauvoir (1952) described as mammalian responsibility. Women who had enjoyed a particularly egalitarian intimate relationship were often surprised and disappointed that once the baby was born, the responsibilities of day-to-day care became her 'job'. Harriet [career woman] explains:

Before he was born I knew just as much about bringing up a tiny little baby as my partner, exactly the same amount, we knew the same amount about pregnancy and everything, but because it was happening to me and the bottom line is that I'm here every day and breastfeeding, I've had to do something to find out some of the answers if possible...

Being at home with the baby proved particularly difficult for many older mothers, especially career women, several of whom had few links to their local community. Prior to the baby's birth, these women seldom spent time home alone and the centrality of work in their lives precluded shopping days or community-based activities, other than on weekends. Lesser achieving and younger women in this study, seemed more connected to the community in which they lived and, indeed, they often continued to live close to where they had grown up. For career women, this strangeness of being at home resulted in a tendency to go out often in the early days, which contributed to a lack of routine and also created dilemmas for the mother when the baby was unsettled. For Abigail [career woman] being 'stuck at home' was a particularly dis-empowering experience:

I think, one of the issues is when you're used to having a project, whether it's your work or ... if you're older used to having you know 'this is my domain, this is my power base' it shifts your power base to the home, I find that very boring, I find it anti intellectual, I don't like the fact that my domain is now the home!

Jeanne [dream-come-true] also felt strange to be at home alone:

In the beginning when I had her I tended to go out a lot and I think, not spending a large amount of time at home ... to be all alone in the house and sort of David working long hours and he works the weekend as well...

117

Generally, this early phase of tumultuous change seemed to abate somewhat at about one month postpartum, consistent with Mercer's (1986) finding of significant transition markers at 1 and 4 months. However, Mercer's later marker at 4 months postpartum is slightly out of kilter with this study's findings. In the following section, the adaptation experiences of the mothers from approximately one to four months postpartum are evaluated. There is, expectedly, some overlap of the mothers' experiences, which do not fall neatly into exact temporal categories.

The struggle 1-4 months

This next stage was characterised by the mothers' dawning awareness of irrevocable life-change and the realisation that the task was a long-standing one. This understanding is similar to that described by Barclay et al. (1997) as "facing the overwhelming process of becoming a mother and the consequences this has on one's life" (p. 722). Participants here described a whole palette of conflicting feelings as they struggled to find a way through the morass of emotion and fatigue that was their experience of new motherhood. Sub themes relating to the 'struggle' include: realising that the task was a long-standing one: ambivalence; issues of self; feeling very unsure, and finally, working through using work strategies. Particular concerns related to the unsettled infant. Each of these sub-themes is discussed in the following section.

Realising that the task was a long standing one

Although for the majority of participants, pregnancy was a much planned and highly sought after state, several women, particularly career women, described feelings of ambivalence in the early days of mothering. This disparity manifested once the initial euphoria of giving birth and the succeeding terror of the first weeks had diminished somewhat and possibly relates to the new mother's first opportunity for thought. It co-existed with the realisation that there was 'no turning back'. An element of grieving for the woman's former life is evident. Interestingly, although many of the mothers felt ambivalence in their early mothering experiences, it was not discussed at the early interviews. It was only later when the mother had achieved a more 'normal' maternal identity and was enjoying her infant, that she felt she could discuss those feelings. Margaret [career woman] explains:

I remember thinking a couple of weeks after Harry was here and I had got him up and I was bathing [him] and I thought I have to do this every day of my life and I'm thinking I don't know if I like it!

Petra [career woman] also found the accommodation difficult:

The biggest adjustment was losing independence I think ... because there've been times when I've just wanted my old life back...

There was an overall element of grieving for the woman's former life, similar to that described by Rubin (1984), though at the same time the women were keen to interject that these feelings did not in any way detract from their feelings of love for the infant. Indeed they were often defensive of this point and eager to assure me that despite the emotional turmoil of their lives, they felt loving and protective towards the infant. In contrast with the findings of this study, Mercer (1986) found that during the first month postpartum, older mothers in her comparative study often expressed frustration and questioned their decision to have a baby (p. 119) and similar struggles are described by younger mothers in other studies, for example, Barclay et al. (1997). In this study, although many of the more accomplished mothers were clearly struggling, there was never any questioning of the decision to have a baby among these women. One possible explanation for this finding may be an unwillingness on the part of the older professional mother to even consider the question of whether or not it was the 'right' decision, when she had invested so much in having a baby. Younger mothers in this study tended to be more forthright in describing the misery of early mothering.

In speaking of the misery of early motherhood, the following interesting phenomenon came to mind. In the early interviews, participants, again usually career women, often expressed the misery of early mothering and, at the end of a long tale of woe and discomfort, punctuated by episodes of such events as bleeding and cracked nipples, expressing milk, painful haemorrhoids and exhaustion, these mothers would finish the conversation with a well worn cliché, such as 'but you'd do anything for them [babies]' or 'but you wouldn't be without them'. It was almost as though they suddenly realised what they had been saying and renounced their former position. At first, I did not know what to make of this incongruity, but it was clearly of some significance and I heard it repeatedly. After discussing it with my panel adviser and thinking about to whom the women were likely to repeat this cliché, I realised that it related to a woman rehearsing her story, as she tried to position herself within her new and as yet ill-fitting maternal identity (Carolan, 2004). This 'rehearsed story' fit with social discourses surrounding motherhood but belied the mental struggles many of the mothers faced. The women's words conformed to prevalent social understandings of motherhood as a wonderful time, and infants as innocent and priceless (Hays, 1996) and parallels can be found in West's (1990) work. In this paper West compares two apparently similar sociological studies of families with disabled children but which resulted in entirely different accounts of their situations. He then discussed the notion of public versus private accounts, where public accounts are understood to be a reproduction of acceptable social meanings and private accounts are understood as "reflecting a private and potentially much less acceptable, reality" (p. 1229). Within the mothering literature, this notion of public versus private accounts is not well addressed though it seems likely that similar forces were at hand in this study. Here, the new mothers I interviewed appeared anxious to convey to me that they were behaving 'normally' and were competent and happy within their new role. This, I believe, was what they understood as socially 'appropriate behaviour' for a new mother. Although notions of truth or reliability are not often associated with the stories people tell, and indeed seem contrary to qualitative valuing of individual stories, nonetheless, the notion of private versus public accounts is a useful one, and provides one framework for understanding the mothers' articulation of seemingly contradictory accounts. Razack (1993) provided another possible explanation. In her article, addressing law and education, she discussed the contradictions of everyday life and the 'multiple nature of subjectivity' (p.62). This, she felt, permitted articulation of multiple and conflicting 'realities'. Therefore, it was, it seemed, possible for participants to harbour two conflicting stories about experiences of mothering at one time. They could indeed have felt both miserable and happy, depending on which discourse they invoked at that time.

Significantly, as discussed in chapter 3, the creation of stories is thought to occur within cultural and social boundaries (Butler 1996; Chase 1995; Davies 1991; Davies & Harre 2001; Gergen 2001; Holstein & Gubrium 2000; Rosenwald & Ochberg 1992; White 1981), meaning that an individual's storytelling is restricted to what is understood/ acceptable within his/her cultural milieu. Analysis of diverse or conflicting stories should thus yield recognizable commonalities, rendering the 'truth' of such accounts of lesser importance than one might suppose.

Ambivalence / my whole life is changing

Several participants found that life changes relating to motherhood far exceeded those imagined. Some mothers reported a certain ambivalence and felt guilty and cheated that they did not like mothering very much. A number questioned if they were indeed 'cut out for the job'. Principal concerns centred on feeling displaced to second place and a lack of predictable routine or order.

Removal to second place

In this study, the problematic removal to second place is described by older mothers exclusively and is more prevalent among the dream-come-true mothers, in contrast to the findings of other studies. Here, Angela [dream-come-true] explains her difficulties:

[It's] not you any more! It's not my husband or myself, it's always Georgia in everything that I do, I have to think of her first.

Although there is little mention of maternal displacement within the 'transition to motherhood' literature, it is not an unknown concept. However, some differences are noted between this study's findings and those articulated elsewhere. Within the literature the notion of maternal displacement seems to be described particularly by well-educated older mothers, in contrast to this study's findings where it was associated principally with less well-educated mothers. For example, Falk (2000) conducted a doctoral study into the subjectivity of mothering, and found that her participants, middle-class, college-educated first-time mothers over 28 years, often described a feeling of conflict at being moved to second place. Similarly, Cudmore (1997) in her doctoral study of primigravidae aged 28-36, found that her participants described surprise at experiencing themselves as secondary to their infants.

It's just so different / wanting a routine

For many participants, particularly women with limited prior exposure to young children, the experience of minimal personal time was problematic. A lack of predictability made planning difficult and mothers, again principally career women, complained of feeling captive to the infant's needs. Making appointments or planning ahead proved particularly problematic. Several mothers responded by trying to work out the baby's routine and organise their day around likely feeding and sleep times, but found it difficult when the baby did not 'fit in'. Kerri [career woman] explains:

But it's just so different ... I always knew that as soon as you had her you would have someone attached to you everywhere you went but there's really no [break] ... if she was

bottle fed it would be different, but I think because she's breastfed she's always with you
and the days are always different ... I think that's what I found really hard at first, I wanted
some sort of routine and I couldn't get it and I'd think 'oh she sleeps at this time, ... and
then all of a sudden she'd change her pattern around ... I make an appointment in advance,
so you think yeah, at the minute she's awake between da da da so I'll make my appointment
at such a time, but by the time I'd reached it, it was always the wrong time or whatever, it's
impossible [despondent].

Dream-come-true mothers tended not to express the same level of concern at disturbing the infant's routine and in general did not try to plan their days to such an extent. Janet [dream-come-true] explains how she works around her infant:

I can do whatever I like, if I want to go out then she just comes with me, the timing might
not be right, you know, things sometimes, ... you might be late.

Young-achievers in this study adopted a similar approach to the dream-come-true mothers and tended to take the baby along when they went out. In general they seemed less troubled than career women about predictable routines. Many had a mother or sister to leave the baby with if needing to attend an appointment. Madeleine [young-achiever] explains her attitude:

I just took her with me wherever I went and I left her bag ready in the boot of the car ... if I
had something important on Mum would take her.

The experience of younger and less accomplished mothers in this study raises the question that younger mothers, or mothers unused to highly structured lives may be more flexible around routines. Although this feeling of being "beholden to the infant" is not exclusively seen among older mothers and indeed is described by Crouch and Manderson (1993), as the first emotional state of motherhood for all mothers (p. 133), it seems particularly salient to the experiences of career women in this study. Midwives from the focus groups postulate that this situation relates to the older mothers having had a much longer time of not feeling obligated to anyone:

They've had it longer too, they've been really well looked after, for 38, 40 years and
they've maintained a lifestyle. Chris [midwife]

At the same time as feeling the need for routine, women in this study frequently described 'wanting to keep something of myself' and not wanting to 'surrender' all sense of the person they had been prior to maternity.

Issues of self / wanting to keep something of myself

This tendency was most commonly displayed by career women and there was a sense that a complete surrender to maternity might have serious implications for the woman's self esteem. Cassie [career woman] explains:

As an older women, I think, I think it's important that you don't lose who you are straight
away, IT'S WHO YOU ARE! ... And I think a little baby who doesn't respond straight away
can be quite demoralising when this is all you do now!

For Rosie, [career woman] witnessing her sister's struggles around maternal adaptation galvanised her own resolve not to surrender herself completely to the chaos of new motherhood:

My sister being at one extreme and me seeing that example ... I was determined not to live
that way, I was determined that my baby would be out of the house the first week!

While Melanie [young-achiever] employed a different approach, insisting on 'time out' when she had had a trying day:

There are times when he's pushed too many buttons and I'll just put him to bed, I'll be
doing something over here and he will have his own space over there.

For many mothers in this study, preservation of self was a concern at this stage and several described 'trying to hold on to who I am', feeling that a complete surrender to maternity would be damaging to the woman's sense of self. This concept manifested in many ways, such as the woman's need to reiterate her personal accomplishments. Indeed, in the early interviews, I became aware of the more

123

professional mother's need to establish with me, that she was a person of some social consequence. On initial contact I collected background detail, such as age, level of education and work history to date. I made it clear that I was collecting it out of demographic interest and in a bid to establish if there were differences in maternal adaptation that related to such variables. I had anticipated a brief paragraph, but many women, particularly more accomplished women, were at pains to provide elaborate detail of their educational and career prowess. It seemed particularly important that I acknowledge their credentials before the interview commenced. Initially, I did not know what to make of this, as to me they were already worthy members of society, though eventually I came to realise it related to issues of self and adaptation. Many women articulated a sense of 'not knowing where they fit' and as well-read and well-educated women they were aware that stay-at-home mothering in advanced societies does not carry the social clout that academic or professional status does (Hoffnung, 1995). Another element of 'wanting to keep something of myself' related to the woman's self-presentation.

Self-presentation

There was a tendency among the better-educated and more professional mothers to attach considerable significance to appearing well groomed and 'in control'. For some, like Harriet [career woman], this was a new experience, as previously she was happy to dress down on the weekend:

> *[Now] even if I'm staying at home during the day, I have to get up, get dressed and put make-up on, whereas before I had a child I didn't do that! ... ... that's important for me! That's just a me thing ... if I was just getting up and putting on an old tracksuit, I think, ... the sort of person I am, that would probably depress me.*

In contrast, less well-educated women were disparaging of such 'self pre-occupation' and did not personally feel the need to keep up appearances. Karine [dream-come-true] explains:

> *I don't have an issue with appearances, I've never been like that ... I think it's bad that some are more of a peacock than others ... if I'm at home I just have my fluffy slippers on.*

Feeling very unsure

Participants also reported feeling really unsure about looking after an infant but nonetheless were keen to 'do things properly' and to 'master' the task of motherhood. The uncertainty of this stage presents as an amelioration of the terror and anxiety of the woman's introduction to mothering. Many of the mothers, again principally career women, worried about their 'adequacy' to the task. Still others were concerned with 'bad habits'. Karen [young-achiever] explains:

You constantly doubt yourself, you constantly go round in circles and then you think am I setting up a bad pattern for life, am I ever going to be able to not have a dummy. [*]

Gayle [career woman], a highly accomplished academic, worried that she might not be equal to the task of stimulating her infant and providing the 'right' environment:

Sometimes, I feel I'm inadequate to the task of playing with her, it's really weird, I feel I'm not qualified enough to do that! ... You're conscious that you have to have activities planned every step of your life...

In this study, a feared inadequacy around infant cognitive stimulation was exclusive to the better-educated mothers and is consistent with the model of 'intensive nurturing' described by Hays (1996) and Hattery (2001), and discussed briefly in chapter 2.

Overall, stages of struggle and adaptation are commonly attributed to new mothers of all ages (Barclay et al., 1997; Falk, 2000; McVeigh, 1997a, 1997b; Pridham & Chang, 1992; Sethi, 1995), however in this study, the experiences of primiparae over 35, particularly career women, seemed very intense and may be related in part to clear role descriptions and structured lifestyles. This stage of adjustment is further discussed in a later section of this chapter. What follows now is the unique approach to mothering favoured by career women of this study.

Working through using work strategies

Once the immediate fears of the infant succumbing had diminished and the new mother had an opportunity to assess the situation, most participants here attempted to 'get to grips' with their circumstances. The more professional women, particularly, then attempted to import work strategies into their mothering experiences and made concerted efforts to 'sort' things out. Indeed, the language used by the more professional women, showed a particular penchant for managerial or business-like problem-solving tactics. Although we will see in the next chapter that this approach ultimately works

---

[*] pacifier

well and the professional mother is resourceful and proactive in accessing information to meet her needs, initially this approach fit poorly within the unpredictable disorder of new mothering and failed to address the complexities and challenges therein. This sub-optimal fit then gave rise to other concerns and distress when carefully formulated plans did not work. For example, one mother had decided that she would work on her computer for blocks of three hours at least twice daily, based on her reading that her newborn infant would most probably sleep for up to 18 hours a day initially. She was distressed to find that her infant was very unsettled and that some days it was impossible to work at all. This, she interpreted as an indication of underlying pathology and many paediatric visits later was still unconvinced of her baby's health.

Others kept inventories of the infant's intake and output amounts and referred to notes taken at the hospital, in a bid to establish a routine and get to grips with the situation. Similar to the approach utilised in pregnancy planning, mothers made plans in possession of the related facts but often without taking the infant's contribution into account. Unexpected, but otherwise normal, events often gave rise to disproportionate concerns. Rachel [career woman] explains:

> *You go by the guidelines in there, virtually! So that's what we did, the 80mls, checked his nappy, no that was fine, gave him his meal, coochy coochy, had a little chat to him, then the squealing started, we tried to burp him and that would've gone on for two hours, more than two hours because we were too frightened to put him down, in case he held his breath and did not wake up or whatever ... he had his arms out all the time, we thought that was making him restless, though we then decided, after the squealing had continued for hours, that we would swaddle him up.*

In the following segment, examples of the managerial type language employed by the more professional women are presented. This language is in stark contrast to the words used by less professional women. Gayle [career woman] explains her mothering approach:

> *I'd always had to organise things at work, coz I ran something so... the skills that were there actually came to the fore a bit with her, I mean they had to...*

Cassie [career woman] shows her understanding of the possible mismatch between work strategies and infant care:

At 35+ you're <u>a troubleshooter</u>, you <u>work problems out</u>, you're in charge of people and all
of a sudden you have a baby that <u>you can't solve!</u>

Throughout the early stages of mothering, the more accomplished women of this study frequently referred to 'doing it properly' and mastering the 'task' of mothering. This theme seems to be underscored by the women's anxiety around 'failing' to live up to expectations.

'Doing it properly' / mastering the 'task'

In this study, the tendency to want to 'do things properly' and to master the task of mothering presents most commonly among career women accounts. Issues of performance seem to drive this notion, which is consistent with other aspects of the women's lives and careers, as discussed in chapter 2. This approach may indeed relate to prevalent work ethics. At this stage, many women described worrying extravagantly about the image they projected. A tendency towards defensiveness is also noted. For example, Sally's [career woman] experience left her very sensitive to perceived criticism of her twins:

You want that perfect image and then put that in to the babies and then if some one makes
a comment ... I remember my mother, she came down a few weeks ago and she said 'oh,
Matthew's looking a bit fat!' and it hasn't left me, you know and its like ohhh she could've
stabbed me that's why I hate it, I know I'm going to stress about it for weeks, how dare they
[criticise] ... all my life I've not been able to take criticism of myself and now all of a
sudden ... the babies ...

This aspect of 'doing it properly' was well recognised by the midwives:

They want things to be perfect, a lot more than other women want them to be ... used to
success ... in whatever area they worked in ...

Jill [midwife]

Della [M&CHN] also showed a clear understanding of the angst the mother felt when things were less than manageable:

If you have a baby that's well behaved and does the right thing, then everything is terrific, but if the baby is difficult then the mother has a very hard time in rationalising, ... she tries to work out why this is happening and she goes into great detail, ... I think ... to try to achieve what it is she's wanting the baby to do. I think they have difficulty in the fact that if their baby is very unsettled etc. etc. they find it very difficult if they don't fit in some sort of routine.

Indeed, an attitude towards conscious, striving mothering receives some attention within the literature. For example, Dally (1982) describes a tendency towards mothering as a conscious activity rather than being informed by "intuition and experience" (p. 123). Barlow and Cairns (1997) additionally discuss maternal adherence to social expectations as contributing to active maternal striving (p. 238). A similar tendency was noted in this study, again among the more educated mothers, some of whom describe the 'chore' or 'task' of mothering. In addition to investing considerable energy in 'doing it properly' women in this study also described a tendency to berate themselves when they slipped up or overlooked some aspect of infant care.

Being hard on myself

This tendency towards self-censure was common among career women particularly, but was also noted among lesser achieving women. Some displayed considerable angst about public appearances or behaviour that they considered negligent, such as forgetting something. In contrast, younger mothers in this study tended to display more pragmatic attitudes. Here Sally [career woman] illustrates her concerns:

You know I went out one day, ... and as usual whenever I go out it's a full on drama when I get out of the house I go oooh! [makes gesture of collapse] ... and I got way up the street and realised that I did not have any blankets for them ... and I thought ... I think will I go back, no I won't have time, I just kept going no one said anything but I kept looking at them and freaking out the whole time! ... I kept saying to myself 'if they get cold, if something happens to them'... it's a horrible feeling, you're so, what's the word, ... I'm so hard on myself, I've always been really hard on myself ... but when I do stuff up I get really hard on myself and it's ridiculous and I just stress myself so badly ...

Jane [career woman] berated herself for behaving irresponsibly when she thought her infant might have a temperature and she had not prepared for such an eventuality:

The other night ... he was laying in my arms, he had little beads of perspiration and I thought 'Oh, my God, he's getting a temperature' and I thought 'I haven't even got a thermometer' in the house. I was really worried about not having a thermometer, I was thinking that in terms of not being prepared and not having a thermometer for him ... I thought that was really irresponsible.

Public performance

In general, performance was very important to professional women, some of whom described worrying considerably about their public appearances. Several spoke of watching other mothers and adjusting their behaviour accordingly. There was a sense of working out what 'appropriate' maternal performance encompassed and mothers then tailored their own performance to 'fit' within social discourses of mothering, similar to that described in chapter 3, as moulding one's behaviour to accepted norms (Foucault, 1988a). Kelly [career woman] explains her concerns:

You're frightened if you are doing the right thing or the wrong thing or whatever ... sort of looking over your shoulder, God, am I doing everything OK? Am I holding him properly, what am I doing? You're very self-conscious about it, I think...

As we will see in a later chapter, new mothers' groups provided one opportunity for participants in this study to observe mothering techniques firsthand. These groups also provided a safe observational environment for women with little prior exposure to infants. In this way, women learnt what was expected of them as mothers.

In the final section of this chapter, the unsettled infant is discussed, as an extension of public performance.

The unsettled infant

The unsettled infant was a cause of great concern, both privately and publicly, and several mothers, principally career women, described going home, abandoning full shopping trolleys or leaving without eating lunch, if the baby was unsettled and difficult to soothe when out. Rachel's [career woman] angst compounded by her concerns to 'avoid bad habits' and to prevent manipulation by the infant, is obvious:

> But at the time, he's shrieking, I was terrified, absolutely terrified of him, that was my biggest fear, the minute he started to cry, not to jump to him straight away, I knew there was nothing wrong with him, but it still troubled me, him being upset ... like I'm not in control, I don't know how to help him.

M&CHNs from the focus groups showed a clear understanding of the career woman's need for the infant to be 'settled':

> Sleeping consumes them, 'how long'... 'Does your baby sleep through'? And when do they sleep through? ... They need the baby to sleep, it's just a real thing, isn't it? So they measure how good a mother they are by how much it sleeps, by how settled their baby is!
> Cathy [M&CHN]

Overall, infant temperament is recognised within the literature as impacting significantly on early mothering experiences for all mothers (Barclay et al., 1997; Drummond, McBride & Wiebe, 1993; Elliot, Drummond & Barnard, 1996; Keefe, Froese-Fretz & Kotzer, 1998; MacArthur et al., 1991; Mercer, 1986; Porter & Hsu, 2003; Rubin, 1984; Twiss, 1989), though once again, there is a paucity of literature pertaining specifically to older mothers. In this study, most mothers experienced distress and concern when the infant cried for prolonged periods. Mercer (1986) understood this tendency well, describing the effect of prolonged crying on the new mother, as resulting in "raised anxiety and feelings of helplessness" (p. 121). Within the limited existing literature there is no clear consensus of how infant fussiness impacts on maternal adaptation among older mothers. Drummond et al. (1993) conducted a qualitative study of 19 mothers in a bid to evaluate maternal understanding of infant crying over time. The participants came from a wide range of socio-economic backgrounds and included both first-time and subsequent mothers, although there is no breakdown of age. Women were interviewed at 6 weeks, 10 weeks and 16 weeks postpartum. Drummond et al. (1993) found that "primiparous mothers accused the infant of psychological reasons for crying at all interview times" (p. 404) and described feeling manipulated by the infant. Meanwhile, Twiss (1989), who conducted a comparative study into the transition experiences of older [over 35] versus younger [20-29] mothers, found infant fussiness to be an indicator of transition difficulty for older, but not for younger, mothers.

In this study, older mothers, irrespective of education, tended to feel personally responsible for any difficulties such as excessive infant crying and would go to enormous lengths to discover 'what they were doing wrong'. There was seldom any suggestion of infant blame and, in general, the women did not recognise infant personality as a contributing factor. A distinctly 'problem orientated' approach to the difficulty of infant crying dominated. This co-existed paradoxically with fears of infant manipulation, which seemed to emanate from outside the woman and were much less prominent than fears of maternal inadequacy. Younger mothers in the current study also expressed concern around the unsettled infant, but were more likely to seek advice from friends and family than to worry how they as mothers were contributing.

Discussion

In general, there is a certain resonance between the early mothering experiences of the current study participants and findings of other studies of maternal transition, particularly the work of Barclay et al. (1997) and Sandelowski (1995a). The principal differences relate to the extent of frustration and angst experienced by the mothers and also to the length of time to maternal adjustment. Older mothers in this study, particularly career women, seemed to travel through the various stages of adjustment at a considerably slower rate and with good deal more angst than mothers in comparable studies of younger / less professional mothers. For example, Barclay et al. (1997) investigated transition to motherhood among 55 new mothers aged 23-39 years in metropolitan Sydney, the majority of whom had worked in clerical / manual occupations. They found that transition to motherhood was mediated by a variety of stages such as feeling 'drained', 'unready' and 'alone' and resolved by 'realising' and 'working it out'. Feelings of loss of sense of self and lifestyle were commonly described. In the current study, participants journeyed along similar pathways, though their experiences were rendered perhaps more intense by struggles and surrender of self, particularly for those women with significant career investment. Nelson (2003a), who studied the experiences of mothers over 30 years, concurred with this view finding a 'planned intensity' among the experiences of older primiparae.

In contrast, Mercer (1986), found little age-related difference in maternal adjustment by four months, reporting that an "identifiable adaptation phase in mothering was evident" (p. 162), at this stage for all age groups. This finding is in contrast with her earlier discussion of poorer maternal adjustment among older mothers at one-month postpartum. Similar to this study, Sandelowski (1995a) who investigated

131

the transition to parenthood for infertile couples, found stages of "struggle and triumph" (p. 123) mediated the participants' journey. Sandelowski further described stages of relinquishing infertility and a re-tailoring of the individual's view of nature. A clearly defined stage of holding back during pregnancy is also discussed, which Sandelowski (1995a) interpreted as a "strategy aimed at self preservation" (p. 127), lest the childbearing outcome be unfavourable. This trend is also reported in Rothman's (1994) pointedly titled 'Tentative Pregnancy', wherein Rothman describes a state of suspended investment in pregnancy related to concerns around fetal abnormality. The following quote illustrates Rothman's understanding-"only after an acceptable judgement has been declared, only after the fetus is deemed worthy of keeping is attachment to begin" (p.114). Sandelowski's findings relate more specifically to participants' experiences of parenthood following a period of infertility and clearly involves a re-alignment of participants' views of normality, nonetheless, similar findings in the current study do not necessarily relate to fertility issues. IVF pregnancies accounted for seven pregnancies among the older participants of the current study, though the process of 'holding back' was described by several mothers, many with natural conceptions. This process appeared to relate to perceptions of being 'at risk' and to having a 'last chance pregnancy'. Women here protected themselves emotionally by keeping busy and not engaging with the pregnancy. Interestingly, among the older participants who had conceived naturally, four had consulted a fertility specialist over the length of time it had taken to conceive and an additional two were to commence fertility treatment within a few months, when they had spontaneously achieved pregnancy. This additional association with sub-fertility may perhaps explain some of the parallels found between this study and Sandelowski's (1995a) study.

Summary

In conclusion, a review of the temporally ordered sequence of transition to motherhood, at 0-4 months postpartum has been attended in this chapter. This stage was characterised to varying degrees, by feelings of anxiety and inadequacy among the participants and a tendency towards vigilance. The 'nightmare' of early parenting (1-4 weeks) is also presented, together with the struggles and ambivalence encountered by many mothers in this study. Although early mothering presents challenges for women of all ages and indeed this stage is frequently described within the literature as a time of dis-equilibrium and upheaval, nonetheless, the experiences of older primiparae, as described here, seem exaggerated. The sequence of transition to motherhood for this group of women also appeared to occur at a slower rate than that reported elsewhere.

Older mothers in this study, particularly professional women, tended to have exacting standards and worried considerably lest they be evaluated as 'not doing things properly'. Self-censure and blame

132

were common among this group and may relate in part to a mismatch of expectations and to fastidious work standards. Major concerns enumerated by the mothers, such as fatigue, concerns with mothering ability and concerns about the infant are common to all new mothers, though again, they seem to present for this group with greater intensity.

Finally, anxiety and perceptions of infant vulnerability, as experienced by many healthy older primiparae and described here by participants, appear to negatively affect the early mothering experiences of this group of women.

In the following chapter, mothering at 4–6 months postpartum is discussed. This stage is characterised by 'giving in / letting go' as the mother comes to 'realise that things work better' if she 'works around the baby'. A series of breakthroughs are also discussed and the mother gains confidence as she 'finds her own way'.

CHAPTER 6
GIVING IN / LETTING GO

They're just like a slug in the beginning, lying there and needing everything, ... now he's giving something to you too and it's good watching him learn things ... just seeing it click and all that, it's just so much fun...

Chapter 6 discusses maternal experiences at 4-6 months postpartum for the study participants. The under-girding theme is that of giving in and letting go, as participants came to realise that their lives were easier when they accommodated infant needs rather than impose maternal routines on the infant. In the early stages of mothering, participants of this study, particularly older professional women, appeared to understand care of the infant as an awesome responsibility, which was accompanied by anxiety and a tendency towards vigilance. This next stage, occurring at 4-6 months, signalled the light at the end of the tunnel. Mothers now spoke of 'getting something back' for all their hard work and in general described this time as a 'turning point'.

This stage was characterised then, to varying degrees, by feelings of discovery and 'breakthroughs' as the mothers came to 'know' their infants and understand their cries. The infant smiled and became more interactive, frequently rewarding the mother's efforts and became a 'little person' rather than the enormous responsibility he/she had been up until this point. Mothers spoke of realising the infant was 'not so fragile' and also of realising that there was no one right way to care for an infant. There was a dawning understanding of having to find one's own way and participants spoke of tailoring their approach to their infant's individual needs and their own personal situation.

The literature relating to transition to motherhood is replete with examples of this stage of realisation, though for the participants of the current study, realisation seemed to occur at a later time than that discussed elsewhere. In general, concerns about the infant and quality of mothering had, by now, diminished and the woman's growing confidence enabled her to sift through proffered advice and make choices. Principal concerns now centred on SIDS, ensuring sufficient sleep and preparation for returning to work. The unsettled infant continued to be problematic for many mothers and a tendency to attempt to 'fix the problem' by attending 'sleep schools' was demonstrated. Finally, the older professional mothers' skills of organisation and information seeking came to the fore at this stage and mothers showed themselves to be pro-active and resourceful in terms of seeking information and assistance.

In this chapter, there are four main areas of attention. Themes of 'giving in / letting go' are explored, together with stages of 'realising', as the mother comes to know her infant. Secondly 'finding my own way' is evaluated as a resolution of the struggles of early parenting. Thirdly, concerns such as infant sleeping patterns and SIDS are evaluated and finally, concerns around socialisation of the infant are discussed. Findings are then compared to current literature.

Introduction

New maternity is commonly considered to be a tumultuous period for primiparous mothers and indeed the literature is replete with examples (Barclay et al., 1997; Falk, 2000; McVeigh, 1997a, 1997b; Pridham & Chang, 1992; Rubin, 1984; Sethi, 1995). Most new mothers experience disruption and adjustment, as they adapt to their maternal roles. Maternal adjustment is considered to be greatest in the first month, but according to Pridham and Chang, "early patterns of regulation are consolidated" by 2-3 months (1992, p. 205) and within the literature most mothers are considered to have adapted by three months postpartum (Mercer, 1986; Pridham & Chang, 1992; Sethi, 1995). The findings of this study however, suggest that maternal adaptation occurs at a considerably slower pace for first-time mothers over 35 years, particularly for those women with advanced careers and limited prior experience of children. A mismatch between maternal expectations and later experience may also contribute. Anxiety-inducing circumstances, such as postpartum complications or infant illness, are discussed in the literature as adding to the disruption of this period (Nelson, 2003b) and, although the associated infants in this study were healthy term infants, participants seemed to have had exaggerated concerns. It may be that maternal anxiety and perceptions of infant vulnerability, common among this study's participants, have contributed to a slower than usual maternal adaptation. Overall, 4-6 months was a significant marker for changes in maternal attitude and role behaviour in this study and is perhaps a little later than Mercer's (1986) finding of a significant marker for transition at 4 months. Here, themes of giving in and letting go presented as a way of moving forward in the transition trajectory.

Giving in (4-6 months)

In this study, 4-6 months postpartum was characterised by a realisation that although it was possible to preserve much of the mothers' prior life, it simply was not 'worth the hassle'. Mothers described realising that life ran more smoothly when the mother 'gave in' and accommodated infant needs, rather than impose maternal routines on the infant. In the early days of mothering, participants expended considerable effort in planning and organising their days. Now there was a surrender to the infant's needs and a change in maternal attitude from adversarial to accommodating and this change was most marked in the accounts of the more professional women. For many mothers, this level of 'surrender' was unanticipated and was preceded by a stage of struggle, as described in the prior chapter. Here, Margaret [career woman] described her dawning realisation that 'blasting through' just was not a good long-term approach:

> *I tried to sort of blast through it in the beginning, just get him in the pram, that's it, we're going walking and it took us, John and myself both, a little while to realise that, like we started to feel like people don't do it! ... and after a while I thought 'why are we doing this'? It's better to when you do need to do things, to do it around him and we're happy to now! ... It took a couple of months [to adjust].*

Letting go because it makes life easier:

'Letting go of things' is also frequently described by the mothers and goes hand in hand with 'giving in'. This stage represented a relinquishing of earlier plans, such as plans to work at home while the infant slept and the mother now adapted her approach to 'doing whatever was necessary'. Once again this sense of surrender was more commonly described by the career women and was scarcely described by the young-achievers, who tended to adopt a more pragmatic approach to change. Abigail [career woman] explains her experience:

> *I know there are some things I have to let go, sometimes that's a bit of a relief but also it's a bit sort of frustrating, a little bit, but what I find hard is that I can't really ... I've actually managed to do a lot of things, but heaps of things that I always used to do have [indicates gone].*

These elements of giving in and letting go are described invariably by the more accomplished older participants and are in contrast to the more balanced approach adopted by younger women. Here Melanie [young-achiever] discusses compromising to accommodate infant needs:

I don't let him keep me in all the time, but if we have a lot of things on I try and have at least one day where we're home all day so he has all of his regular naps and the other couple of days if he misses a nap, well, ok I'll just wear that, so you really do a lot of balancing off with yourself.

The surrender

Overall, career woman accounts are replete with phrases of surrender and many are tinged with regret. The phrases: 'giving in'; 'no choice'; 'having to do it' and 'having to change', appear frequently. Margaret [career woman] explains coming to terms with having 'no choice':

It really reduces you to the basics whether you want to or not, like there's no choice about it and that actually was a bit of a changing point, too, that giving in, when I realised you just have to give in to it ... if we had to sit here all day and he needed to be cuddled by me and fed all day, then I had to do it! At first I thought, no, I can't, we'll go and do other things, ... [now] you realise that's going to be one of those days today!

For Gayle [career woman] the 'surrender' to her daughter's routine was undeniably tinged with regret. Her angst at the loss of spontaneity in her life is balanced by her understanding of the importance of routine:

We've had to change, there's no doubt about that! I mean ... I think you lose the spontaneity of everything, I think that's what's so difficult, you can't just say let's go for a drive ... I can deal with it now, because I know she has to have a routine and I've had to deal with a lack of routine ... I knew, I just knew that it was going to have all these effects, but I must say the first day that someone said to me, now, she has to be in bed by 6.30 / 7 or something like that and this is the maternal nurse [M&CHN] and you have this routine of food, story, bed and you know, I said 'what, you mean we can't go out?' Up till then we were taking Tina out, you could go out and she didn't know what time it was...

A different way of thinking

For many of the career women, this stage of realisation and surrender is accompanied by an understanding that a change in maternal thinking is required. For Jeanne [dream-come-true], a completely different approach to her day was required:

> *I've had to change my times around! [Laughter] it just completely changes your day, you try to get into a different pattern, a different way of thinking, you had to change your thinking.*

Petra [career woman] described changing from doing it her way to accommodating the infant:

> *I think in the beginning I was inclined to try to force him into your [sic] ... way of thinking, but then you realise 'no, you can't do that'! You've got to go into his ways and work around him, it was, just so difficult, you think, 'oh you should be able to do this.'*

One day at a time

One approach adopted by mothers here was to simply live one day at a time, as they came to grips with their situation. Sally [career woman] describes living in the present, rather than making elaborate long term plans. This changed approach to living allowed her to concentrate on 'just getting through' from day to day:

> *It's the first-time I have ever really lived in the present, in my life! Really now, at this moment, not this week or whatever, very much now! ... It's odd, now I'm back working I have people saying 'next week blah, blah, blah can you do this? And I go oh! [gasp] and I find it really hard to make that decision and I'm really terrible with what's gone, you know like... from where I was, I used to have my life sorted out ... now I can't possibly think ahead ... it just happened, that's just the weird thing, it's like it happened and I had no control over that, its all that I could cope with...*

Willing to change

While for most of the career women, restrictions on outings and social activities represented something of a dilemma, some, such as Jane [career woman] were happy to stay-at-home with their infants:

138

Well, I waited this long for my child, I don't want to pass him off to other people because we chose to have a child and I would like to, you know, have the child and not send him off to this, or that ... like it was in a sense, a little bit hard coming to terms with that, you know, but our choice is not to do it, its much more fun being with Keegan than going anywhere ... all these movies come out so quickly on video now, that it doesn't really matter, but I guess I don't find too much of it too hard.

In contrast to a percentage of 'career women', going out to restaurants without the infant presented no dilemma for many of the 'dream-come-true' mothers. Janet summed up her experience as follows:

I thought that was the idea of going out to a restaurant ... [laughing] ... to get away from the baby ... why would you want to bring her?

One possible explanation for this differing degree of struggle and surrender voiced by the career women compared to dream-come-true mothers, may relate to a perceived lack of control. Professional women, used to autonomy and decision making at work may find it difficult to surrender to the whims of infant needs. Based on their reading and discussion with friends, many women in this study, particularly career women, had anticipated that caring for an infant was simply a matter of good time management strategies. These mothers expected to make choices about feeding and sleeping schedules and planned to institute 'good routines' early in their maternal experience. Most had not envisaged the time-consuming demands of newborn care and had made little allowance for infant contribution. In contrast, women from the young-achievers group tended to adopt a more pragmatic approach to accommodating change and did not in general discuss relinquishing their will to the infant's needs. In addition to a surrender to the infants' needs, several of the more accomplished mothers expressed surprise at finding themselves willing to concede earlier career plans or ambitions, despite having a clear life trajectory prior to the infant's birth. This manifested in a return to work at a time later than that anticipated or a negotiation with employers to return to reduced hours and this is considered in more depth in chapter 7. The surprise Rosie felt at realising that she was willing to relinquish her clearly laid out goals is evident in her account:

I guess the other big thing is the anxiety for someone else, I never felt that before and kind of giving up your own life and goals, not personality, but your own life and goals ... I'm willing to give it up, whereas I wouldn't... [have been before].

In general, stages of struggle and resolution are frequently described in the literature surrounding new motherhood. Miller and Sollie (1980) who studied the natural stresses endured by first-time parents (n = 120), found that mothers reported increased levels of personal stress in the early days of parenting, which they later resolved as mothering became more familiar. Sethi (1995), in her narrative study (n = 15) found that mothers experienced tensions while dealing with the "contradictory nature of the processes during the first three months postpartum" and also that many women described feeling "stretched and strained" (p. 236). This stage was followed by a stage of maternal redefinition and adaptation to the mother's new circumstances. Barclay et al. (1997) also described stages of feeling alone and drained prior to reaching a stage of realising and Barlow and Cairns (1997), considered the psychological experience of mothering for 11 participants. They found that mothers described reaching a personal crisis, as "a kind of identity disintegration which threatened their sense of self" (p. 241). This 'crisis' appeared to relate to maternal struggles to balance their own needs and the needs of the child. Resolution of the crisis involved the development of "self-constructed mothering" (Barlow & Cairns, 1997, p. 242) similar to the theme of 'finding my own way' described in this study. Finally, Sandelowski (1995a) described stages of "struggle and triumph" (p. 123) during the transition to parenthood experiences of infertile couples and, although her findings relate to relinquishing infertility prior to moving forward, certain parallels can be found in this study, particularly in relation to struggle and resolution. Indeed, stages of struggle and resolution are well described within the literature, as above, and notions of maternal sacrifice are similarly well attended (Hays, 1996; Rubenstein, 1998; Thurer, 1994), but this sense of 'giving in' and 'letting go' and thus surrendering to infant needs, *per se*, do not receive specific attention.

Realising

For the participants of this study, stages of giving in and letting go were mediated by a series of realisations, such as: realising that the infant was not so fragile; realising it was OK to have negative feelings; realising that it was not possible to 'do it all'; realising 'I could do it' and finally, realising there was no one right way to care for an infant. Stages of realising are common to most new mothers and are especially well described by Barclay et al. (1997), though again, realisation seems to occur at a later stage for the older participants of this study, irrespective of educational status. It seems reasonable to postulate that limited prior exposure to infants and a tendency to be removed from one's natal family may have contributed to this slower than usual understanding of the requirements and responsibilities of infant care. Gayle [career woman] was surprised that the transition took longer than the expected three months:

I think, you have to expect that there's going to be hitches on all fronts for a while, I think it takes at least up to nine months, I mean, we said this is going to be a really hard 12 weeks here, that's what we said to ourselves at the beginning, well it turned out that we were right out with that, we had a concept that ... there would be a period of time, well, I reckon only now some things are working themselves back out again. I think it takes a good nine months to get it sorted, all the bits and pieces.

Realising that the infant was not so fragile

For many of the mothers, realising that the infant was not as fragile as they had previously imagined, was something of a turning point. An associated reduction in anxiety allowed them space to relax a little when handling the baby. Kelly [career woman] explains:

I guess a lot of it was that all of a sudden you just realise it's just a baby, I'm not treating it like a china doll anymore, ... suddenly you just pick him up and throw him into the cot [you] get more confident and you just think 'gee, I'm getting better at this!

Often the infant's father facilitated this growing understanding, as described by Petra [career woman]:

Now we pick him and throw him round and I've found, coz I was quite gentle with him and Mark is quite rough with him and he loves it and I think it was the feeling of confidence from that roughness from Dad that helped me, that I'm not going to damage him too much.

Often, mothers learnt from watching other mothers, at the supermarket, at health centres, parks and within the safety of the M&CHN run 'new mothers' groups' (Carolan, in press- b), as discussed in chapter 7.

Realising it was OK to have negative feelings

Realising that it was OK to have negative feelings around the baby and the associated life changes also proved a turning point for many women. This realisation allowed the woman to address her negative self-talk and recognise the normality of adjustment issues. Petra's [career woman] humorous account illustrates it nicely:

> *And realising it's OK to realise you want to kill them, you just can't follow through [Laughter], there are times when you want to do it, but you just can't [Laughter] there are days when I'm just dying for him [husband] to get home and to hand him [baby] over because its full on all day and there's some days where I'm fine ... one day I opened the door and said 'here's your son!' [Laughter] I'd had a bad day! [laughter laughter] and then you get over that and then you feel guilty that you've had those thoughts.*

For Jennifer [dream-come-true] recognising that it was normal to have feelings of anger and hate towards her infant, on occasion, allowed her the space to work through her emotions:

> *You can be overcome with this terrible guilt but there are times when you really, it's in anger, it's in frustration, but knowing that you have those feelings [of hate], recognising it [as normal] ... I think most women, 90% of women suffer with some sort of depression after they've had their baby.*

Realising you just can't 'do it all'

For several of the older mothers, irrespective of educational status, the early days of mothering were fraught with self-imposed pressure to maintain exacting standards of housework, attend to infant care and comply with the social discourses which dictate that women can 'do it all', as discussed briefly in chapter 2. The women in this study describe reaching a stage of realising that the 'stereotypical mother' was a myth and that not only was it OK not to do everything 'perfectly', but it was simply not possible. This stage of realising allowed mothers to be less self-critical of their performance. For Harriet [career woman], realising that she was not 'superwoman' was something of a turning point:

> *I think that some of the people that wrote about the feminists have now sort of retracted some of the things they said ... well you can't be superwoman! I don't believe you can.*

Janet [dream-come-true] felt it important to ground herself and her expectations on a regular basis:

I know that you have to keep your eye on it [self criticism] as much as possible, but you're not wonder woman and you're not ... I've still got the sheet [you can't do it all] that we got from the health centre and if I feel like I'm getting stressed I read that!

Realising I could do it

For some, realising that they were capable of caring for their infant represented a defining moment in their mothering experiences. Rosie [career woman] explains:

I think a real turning point was when my mother-in-law moved ... we had worked out a system where she [baby] never cried, ... my mother-in-law would come with me in the car and so we always had someone, so she [baby] didn't cry, ... she'd hold her while I got the pram and I thought 'how am I going to do this?' and when she left it was so liberating! If I had realised it, I might have tried it before hand!

Realising that there was no one right way

Realising that there was no one right way of caring for an infant also represented a critical moment for many of the mothers. Extensive reading had left several women with the impression of a limited opportunity to 'get it right' and possible dire consequences of missing cues, such as inadvertently damaging the infant, or establishing 'bad' sleep or feeding habits. Discovering, often through interaction with other mothers at the M&CHN groups, that there was no one 'right' way to care for an infant helped the new mother to find her own way. Petra [career woman] explains:

And I suppose it was more realising that there was no right or wrong way, as well ... and because what works for one doesn't work for another and I think that's the best thing when you're still having the mother' group and knowing what other people have gone through and how they've handled it ... when you don't know if you're doing the right thing, that was, I think that was the most frustrating.

Realising that there was not only 'one way' allowed the women to sort through the various information available and to try out different ways of dealing with new situations and difficulties. Through adopting a trial-and-error based approach, the new mother discovered her 'own way' to care for her infant. This stage of finding one's own way is addressed in the next section.

Finding my own way

'Finding my own way' is one of the five interweaving themes described in chapter 3 and plays an important part in the transition to motherhood experiences of older mothers in this study, particularly career women. Until this stage, mothers had concentrated their efforts on 'doing things properly' and embraced common social discourses around mothering. This adherence to social expectations of mothering prior to finding their own way is similar to what Barlow and Cairn's (1997) describe as a "loyalty to societal expectations" (p. 238) prior to discovering 'self constructed mothering' (p. 241).

Furthermore, before birth, infant care was often understood by the mothers of this study as a matter of good time management. Now there was a growing understanding that the 'one size fits all' approach simply did not address the individuality of mother infant dyads. Margaret's [career woman] account presents a good example. Prior to her infant's birth, Margaret had been at odds to understand how some new mothers were unable to find time to shower and dress before midday. She was therefore surprised to have a similar experience herself, but as time went on, found ways to 'get around it':

> *I used to wonder how on earth people stayed in their pyjamas until lunchtime and it was happening to me every day [laughter] but then you just start to get a few ways to get around it, like now, I just get out of bed and get dressed, because then I feel better about it. I feel like I'm human, instead of thinking 'how come this is happening to me?*

Several mothers expended considerable effort on developing strategies to 'cope' with the disorder of early parenting and to have contingency plans in the event of initial plan failure. This approach is in stark contrast to the more relaxed approach of the 'dream-come-true' mothers. Gayle [career woman] explains her attitude:

> *The best bit of advice that I got from my friend was when she said to me to get through this you have got to have strategies.*

For Annie [dream-come-true], strategies never entered the equation:

I didn't really have a lot of expectations really, ... I took things as they came ... I just go with the flow, if we eat tea at 8.30 we do! [philosophically].

Making sense of the information

The ability to decipher and make sense of the available information represented another major milestone in the transition to motherhood and is closely linked to increasing maternal confidence and finding 'my own way'. Initial efforts to take 'everything on board' are abandoned in favour of selection of advice suitable to maternal requirements and personality. Petra's [career woman] experience is typical:

You got little bits that helped from everyone, not one person, sort of thing, like that particular person had specific ideas but this little bit was good here and that little bit was good there and like the health nurse and that was very helpful and eased your mind about a lot of things. You could call up and ask questions and all that sort of stuff, 'ohh, is this supposed to happen?'

The tendency to take on board all proffered advice was not exercised exclusively by career women in this study, but it was however, more pronounced among that group. In general, dream-come-true mothers tended to be more discriminating and sifted through advice from an early stage, basing their selection on the opinion they held of the person offering advice. Annie explains:

From when he was about 2 months old everyone said if he was crying that it was teething ... that's the thing, everyone becomes an expert! But it depends who it [advice] came from, some people I just thought 'yeah, yeah yeah! And it just went straight in one ear and out the other and other people I'd think 'well, I really respect what she says so I would think about that one.'

Women from the 'young-achievers group' seemed to be positioned somewhere in between, though again they were more likely to have read a considerable amount of literature and to be concerned with making choices. Anita found she decided to go with whichever suggestion made more sense:

145

It's like the other day my Mum was saying 'oh she's hungry, she's hungry' and I asked my other sister, who's a nurse, who's got 2 kids and she said' no, they like the sucking motion and you can't keep feeding them, if you keep feeding them irregular hours then they're going to expect to feed all hours, the doctor said do 3-4 [hours] so I said to Mum, OK I'm not going to feed her, she's not hungry! and she said OK you decide, whatever you think, she got annoyed of course [laughter] I said 'no, I'm going to go by what Dana said, what she said to me made a bit more sense and that's the way I work through it.

Interestingly, although most mothers had achieved this stage of confident decision making by 4-6 months, it was not an exclusive achievement. Gayle [career woman], who had returned to work at approximately 3 months was still clearly struggling at 6 months postpartum. She describes an agony of indecision and misery, and her insecurity around decision-making seemed to make her very vulnerable to suggestion. Here, she describes following her friend's advice, about not allowing her infant to sleep in the parental bed, though it is obvious that she was very unclear about her decision to do so:

She said 'please don't do what we did' and she's the one that put me all into a panic, but she admitted that she had taken her into bed and ... you see, I could've done that and taken her into bed, but I didn't, I thought, I'm going to stand here and persevere in the cold [in the baby's room, where the heating vent is closed due to worries over SIDS] I tortured myself instead. So long as she's not removed from us and thinks we're strange people... [unfeeling]

For most of the participants 'finding my own way' represented a turning point in the transition to motherhood. Until this time the new mother did not have a framework to make sense of the information she accessed, or a knowledge base to support confident decision-making. This situation of ease of access to medical and advanced literature particularly on the Internet, without an accompanying framework to make sense of the information appears to contribute to maternal concerns. Limited family or peer support also seems to have contributed to a slower than usual attainment of decision-making confidence among study participants.

Within the literature, the theme 'finding my own way' is not abundantly addressed, though some references are found. Barlow and Cairns (1997) discuss a loss of "personal identity as the catalyst for

146

the development of self-constructed mothering" (p. 241) and Barclay et al. (1997) discussed a category of 'working it out' as mothers developed skills and gained confidence. Mercer (1986) meanwhile, discussed maternal role adaptation as occurring around four months postpartum and this transition is portrayed as a relatively seamless and unproblematic event for most women. Other authors, such as Sethi (1995), describe a redefinition of self and an acceptance of the baby as a turning point. Additionally, Barlow and Cairns (1997) reported that traditional views of childrearing were often viewed as incompatible with personal philosophies (p. 239) leading to a re-negotiation of life goals. In the following section, a series of breakthroughs are described as the mother comes to 'know her infant' and recognise its cues. Increasing confidence in turn facilitates decision-making.

Breakthroughs / getting to know the baby

At around 3-4 months, most mothers described recognising infant cues and understanding infant crying as purposive. This stage of getting to know the baby and to appreciate its uniqueness was something of a surprise to the older mothers in this study and little difference is noted between the experiences of dream-come-true and career woman mothers. Earlier in the parenting experience, most mothers had used long complicated lists to make sense of infant crying. Soothing involved the use of wide-ranging interventions and each time the infant cried the mother would go through her list in a bid to discover 'what was wrong'. Each episode of crying was understood as constituting a problem. Now, at around 4 months, the mothers describe a dawning understanding of infant crying. There are episodes of breakthroughs similar to the one described below. Annie [dream-come-true] describes her experience:

I remember one morning, he'd had his bottle and I'd put him down on the floor and he was a bit grizzly and I thought 'I wonder what's wrong' so I picked him up and he cuddled in and he went to sleep and I thought 'Ahh' ... so I popped him into bed and he slept for a little while and then next morning, probably about an hour later again he got the grizzly noise going and I thought 'that's tired'! You know, he wants to go to bed ... it was just straight away, bang he was asleep yeah and that grizzle, yeah, I knew that was I'm tired, I want to go to bed, that was just so exciting, that was really good.

For several mothers, recognising the tired infant presented great difficulty initially and they would attempt to distract the perceivably 'grumpy' infant. Frequently they would try a whole range of options to 'sort' out the infant's fussiness. The discovery that the infant was tired often came as a major surprise. Jeanne [dream-come-true] explains:

She was 3 months old before I realised she's tired, my godfather! She's tired! Oh God [laughter] and here I thought she was grumpy or hungry.

Although, generally speaking, mothers at 4-6 months describe understanding their infants' cries as purposeful and as relating mostly to hunger or tiredness, for some there appeared to be a time lag in reaching this stage of interpretation. At 6 months, Jennifer [dream-come-true] still struggled, particularly with night-time crying:

Except in the middle of the night when you go through the list! And you panic and you think 'what could it be?' but then you get the lack of confidence for the small thing, do I give her Panadol? And how much? Am I [over] dosing my child? What happens if it's not teeth? What happens if I'm reading it wrong?' It's not easy at times!

This finding of slower than usual understanding of infant crying is not well addressed in the literature. Drummond et al. (1993), who conducted a qualitative study of 19 mothers, of mixed parity, found that for primiparous mothers, infant crying at 10 weeks was generally viewed as a means of communication and as being associated with hunger and tiredness. By 16 weeks the cry was "determined as a definite communication" (p. 401). Although there is no breakdown of maternal age in this study, given Drummond's interest in adolescent mothers, it is reasonable to speculate that this study may relate to younger women. Within the literature, there is a general understanding of crying among firstborn infants as especially distressing for mothers (van der Wal, van den Boom, Pauw-Plomp & de Jonge, 1998), although maternal understanding of infant crying is not well addressed. St James-Roberts, Conroy and Wishler (1996) discovered that although firstborn infants do not cry substantially more than subsequent infants, first-time mothers were particularly affected by infant crying, though no age-related effects are postulated. In this study, while infant crying was viewed as signalling distress, there was little maternal understanding of cause and mothers reported 'going through their list' of possible causes each time the infant cried. This finding was prominent among all the older mothers and particularly prevalent among the more anxious mothers. It presented to a lesser extent in the 'young-achievers' group.

'Things getting easier'

For most, there was a clearly recognisable stage of things getting easier, as the infant became more settled at night and the mother became more confident and found ways to get around difficulties. Petra [career woman] explains:

It started to get a lot easier, well, not easier but better ... and you felt a bit more in control.

And Gayle [career woman] describes her experience:

I'm amazed that I can actually make food at night, that I can think and actually make meals rather than rely on this catering place that I used to get meals for $8 each. I think that's been a bit of a breakthrough and I thought well she's a bit easier to manage, Mark can do things she's not so dependent on breast milk from me all the time and once you get through that it makes it easy.

Overall, there was a general impression of 'things improving' as the newborn stage gave way to the more responsive infant. Although, in general, increasing maternal confidence was the forerunner of a more relaxed and flexible approach to mothering, it was not a unanimous experience. On one occasion, well after data collection had ceased, one of the study mothers took, her by now 18-month-old toddler, to visit me at the hospital and had insisted on making an appointment time. When the appointment time arrived, I received a phone call from the hospital car park to say that the toddler was asleep and the mother would come up to visit when her daughter awoke. She arrived some 45 minutes later. So surprised were my colleagues, themselves all mothers, that this situation was the source of ongoing discussion and debate for some considerable time. We all wondered at how this mother had become so captive to her baby's routines.

In addition to things getting easier, at this stage, the more professional mothers' organisational skills come to the fore, as discussed below.

Skills I can draw on

Generally speaking, career women, despite having a shaky start, now identified themselves as resourceful and confident in terms of problem solving. Their organisational skills and work experiences seemed to equip them well to deal with childcare dilemmas and decision-making. Sally [career woman] explains:

I would just go to plan B. It depends on what you do for a living, but I've been a project manager for many years and we always come up with problems and hiccups and you get over them, so fortunately, that's my background, so if there's a hiccup, that's OK, that happens so what are my other options, my options are this so let's see if we can do that.

Cassie [career woman] felt that her work experiences equipped her well for caring for her twin boys:

A couple of years ago I was a systems manager and I had up to about 20 programmers under me, you know, various projects and the programmers were all sort of under the age of 25 and I thought they were going to give me a really hard time they were all boys, couldn't be any harder than what I'm about to do because they're all children and on top of that they were programmers, egos and all of that! I remember going around doing my rounds and you'd walk up behind them and you'd think. This is so and so. Everyone had to be treated in a different way! So I was thinking I had a really good grounding.

Maternal and child health nurses from the focus group also recognised the skills many career women possessed and did not necessarily subscribe to stereotypical ideas of older mothering [Appendix C]. Della explains:

They often have lots of skills they can draw on ... there is a bit of a stereotypical idea of what older first-time mothers are like, but I've had first-time elderly mothers that have been completely different, some have been fantastic, others that have been extremely anxious.

Within the scant literature where this theme of maternal work-related skills is addressed, most favour a positive view. Froman and Owen (1989) found a mother's age to be positively related to confidence in infant care activities. Berryman (1991) concurred with this view, claiming "the evidence suggests that older mothers may have skills as a result of their greater maturity which they can contribute to their abilities as a parent." (p. 118). Similarly, Dobrzykowski and Stern (2003) found that older mothers were better able to solve problems because of their "maturity and experience" (p. 251) and also that they were 'street smart' in that they knew how to access resources. Pridham and Chang (1992) considered maternal age and problem-solving abilities to be positively linked (p. 213) and Gottesman (1992) found high levels of competency among older mothers.

In contrast, Mercer (1986) found a lower evaluation of parenting competence among primiparae and more highly educated women and MacArthur et al. (1991), discussed older primiparity as a predictor for depression and anxiety. Twiss (1989), in her doctoral study, found infant fussiness to be an indicator of transition difficulty for older but not younger mothers. Finally, Rubin (1967b) felt that career mothers approached role conflict differently, through either expanding the role and attempting to do everything, which had a tendency to be counter-productive and lead to burnout and distress, or, as the participants of this study largely describe, redefining the role to reduce expectations and accommodate change.

At this stage, most women spoke of enjoying their mothering experiences and describe getting something back for all their hard work. In the early stages of mothering there was a tendency to regard caring for the infant as an 'awesome responsibility' which abated only when the mother started to think of her infant as a 'little person'.

The little person emerges

At around 3-4 months, the infant became increasingly responsive, smiling and interacting with his/her mother, and mothers become aware of the infant as a little person. Kelly [career woman] explains:

At some stage they do become more than a baby, showing more human type behaviour rather than just crying, looking at their hands, recognition, all that!

This recognition of the infant as a little person seems especially delayed among many of the older professional women in this study and may relate to a late 'claiming of the infant'. Rubin first described maternal attachment as the result of a claiming process, during which the mother, in the early neonatal period, ascertains that her infant is normal and whole. The newborn infant is examined and features, such as the shape of the nose and ears, are contrasted with similar features of the father, mother and relatives (Rubin, 1984). This linking of features and behaviours to persons within the family allows the mother to claim the child as belonging to her and the family.

151

In the current study, this process of claiming was highly visible among the lesser achieving mothers and also the younger mothers, who in general had a high degree of family and grandparent contact. Their accounts are replete with examples of speculation about who the infant 'takes after'. Among the career women, this 'claiming' is not quite so visible initially and it may be that the absence of family support and geographical or temporal distance from the older mothers' natal family contributes to this slower than usual claiming of the infant and therefore the slower than usual recognition of the infant as 'human' or as belonging to the family. By approximately 4 months of age most women describe seeing the infant as a 'little person' and, as the infant becomes increasingly responsive and engaging, mothers describe getting something back for all their hard work.

Getting something back

For Sally [career woman] this stage marked a departure from merely going through care routines. Mothers now spoke of getting 'rewards' for their efforts, as the infant smiled and became more responsive:

> *I suppose you feel it's more interactive than, as opposed to just you going through the motions, which you do and a reward, you're getting a reward for it! I can remember certainly, around that stage saying, you know, when my husband came home, saying 'oh such and such did this today!*

For many of the mothers this stage was one of pleasurable discovery, made all the more pleasurable because it was unanticipated. Women spoke of falling in love with their infants as they got to know them. For Petra [career woman], her pleasure in her infant far exceeded her expectations:

> *I think the interaction that you're getting now is heaps better than you could possibly expect ... the bond that you create there, ... you just can't explain that to anyone! It's something you've just got to feel and experience and I think that's heaps better than what I thought it would be ... that cute little smile and giggle.*

Kerri [career woman] was surprised at how different her experience with her infant was compared to experiences she had had with other children:

I think although I've had a lot of contact with babies, sometimes I get the feeling that she knows me so well ... it just amazes me that she knows both of us ... She will smile for us when she won't smile for other people, you know, she chats away when she's with us ... and I can never get that reward with other people's children.

Feeling special

Finding themselves loved and wanted by their infant was a serendipitous experience for many of the women in this study, particularly for 'career women' and this trend is presented here as an extension of 'getting something back'. For the career women in this study, primary motivation for having a baby related to feeling it was the right thing to do, the next thing on their list and finally, a life experience not to be missed. Discovering that the infant loved them and responded to them particularly came as a surprising bonus. Kerri [career woman] explains feeling awed to discover her infant knew and preferred her over others, even 'experienced' family members:

Its amazing, you don't sort of realise ... I didn't realise that you don't really get that response from other children, like if they're crying and you give them back to their Mum ... if she's crying and someone gives her to me she'll stop ... when she [Kerri's baby] came back to me and she stopped crying for the very first time I sort of thought 'oh wow!

Indeed, Kerri went on to describe how she did not entirely believe that her infant preferred her above more experienced others, so much so that she tested it out again at the next family function she attended. Again, her infant was unsettled and crying when Kerri's sister held her, but was easily soothed by her mother. Interestingly, this situation doesn't seem to exist with either the young-achievers or the dream-come-true groups. One possible explanation is that younger women are perhaps not quite so distant temporally from experiences of family and children. Also, among the dream-come-true mothers, in wanting a baby, they had expected to love their infant and to be loved in return and this tendency most probably contributed to maternal confidence and a lack of surprise to discover that the infant preferred them to others.

In general, though this stage of transition represented a time of breakthroughs and lessening burdens, there was also a sense of simmering resentment expressed by many of the women, particularly related to their partner's unchanging life, in the midst of their own irrevocably changed circumstances.

'His things are taken for granted and mine can be arranged'

Despite expectations that it would be a shared experience, many mothers, again particularly career women, found that the baby essentially became their 'job' as briefly mentioned in chapter 5. While the spouse continued to play sport or stay late at work, the new mother found she had to negotiate to have time off. Perceptions of under-appreciated maternal effort were also common and several women described feeling undervalued in their stay-at-home role. Rosie [career woman] explains:

> *And I think sometimes he didn't have enough respect that I was doing enough, he'd say that he was working, I'm not working ...whereas I work more than he did, because he went to gym whereas I had to ask 'can you take care of her while I go somewhere? He didn't ask! ... OK, you work and I take care of her during the day, but then when you come home, I see it as our job and you have no more right to go to the gym than I have to go somewhere else without working it out ... his things are taken for granted and mine can be arranged!*

Concerns

At 4-6 months postpartum, worries and concerns voiced by participants were far less expansive than formerly, encompassing mainly, sleep concerns and SIDS. Secondary worries include: social issues such as 'how we will develop as a family' and worries about 'finding the right balance' between work and family commitments, while still preserving some modicum of selfhood. The principal concerns are ordered here by level of reporting.

Infant sleeping patterns

Infant sleeping patterns were a major source of concern to mothers already returned to work and also to women planning a return to work in the near future. For women with very exacting professions the fragile balance depended largely on the infant sleeping at night, with little room for infant variability. Any change in sleeping patterns was viewed as something of a disaster. Gayle, [career woman] for example, describes her infant's occasional restless night or early rising as a major source of angst:

> *You see, if Tina starts to wake up early, like 6.30 or something, we will have chaos, if she wakes up about 8 ish, that works in ok, but there's been a couple of times with teeth, where she was waking up at about 5.30 and wanting more food and so I would have to feed her*

and then I would have to get her up again about 8 to take her [to childcare] and I was trying to stick to the 8 routine you know, if she starts waking up much earlier then chaos will reign.

In order to prevent infant sleep disturbances, some mothers went to extravagant lengths to reduce likely stimuli or physical causes. Here Gayle describes removing her daughter's activity centre and toys from her cot, in the hope of promoting more settled nights:

We haven't got anything [toys] in the cot at the moment. At one point I took them out coz I thought it might stimulate her. That was one thing I got in the middle of the night... then we took the mobile down because she recently started to grab things and I thought she might pull it down...

But nonetheless feels guilty and defensive about her choices:

Everyone says 'oh we had our baby in the bed with us' but all the books say not to do that.... [reflective], we don't want to do this, because we don't know where it'll lead, we could have her in our bed until she was 5 or something, you just don't know!

For others, poor night-time sleeping was understood as related to the infant's 'nature'. Harriet [career woman] felt her infant's poor sleeping patterns related to his 'stubborn' nature:

And that's his personality he's definitely going to be [indicates stubborn], we're going to have a few battles of will he says I'm not going to sleep, until you actually feel sorry for me and pick me up and cuddle me to sleep ... he's so stubborn, that's what his problem is actually!

Sleep schools and controlled crying

By 4-6 months, the unsettled infant was frequently regarded as problematic for study participants, particularly older mothers. This represents a departure from maternal focus on coping with the needs of a newborn. Now, there was an expectation that the infant should be sleeping at night. Failure of the infant to comply with these expectations was met with a maternal tendency to attempt to 'fix the

155

problem' and mothers report attending 'sleep schools' or 'clinics' in order to teach their infant to sleep through at night. Indeed, sleep clinics have come into prominence in the last five to ten years, largely in response to growing demand by professional women and most of these clinics endorse 'control crying'[20] as a sleep 'training' method. Although the use of sleep schools or controlled crying was not exclusive to career women in this study, the practice was considerably more prevalent among their ranks. All older mothers in this study, irrespective of career investment or level of education, made serious efforts to redress perceived infant sleep deficiencies though both young-achievers and dream-come-true mothers were less likely to attend sleep centres, or use behavioural training to address sleep deficiencies. This differing approach may relate to different levels of career investment between the two groups of older mothers and also to the tendency for the career women to return to work at an earlier stage than their less accomplished sisters. Younger women in this study seemed more accepting of infant-related sleep disturbances. Anthea's [career woman] story of attending sleep school is typical, though at 6 weeks, her attendance is considerably earlier than usual:

> I went to one of those sleep schools at 6 weeks and that was great! I think every mother should go! ... For one day and then back a week later for a day, they give you a week in between, they call it day stay program ... one of the other Mums [mothers' group] just went to Massada for a week because her baby was waking up 3 and 4 times a night at 6 months old. She was in tears, of course, she was exhausted ... honestly, I know I'd be a wreck from the lack of sleep.

Several others attempted to sort the 'problem' out themselves, using 'controlled crying'. Harriet's [career woman] experience is pretty much representative:

> I've got the books and it says you let them cry for 2 minutes then you go back and then four ... and the other thing is that if you want to maintain any sort of life, they're expecting you to stay home every day, to get a routine ... serious routine ... he needs sleep school except I can't bring myself to go to sleep school! I wouldn't be able to cope with it.

---

[20] Control crying is a behavioural training method (Ferber 1987, 1999) whereby an infant is 'taught' to settle him/herself to sleep. The crying infant is attended by the mother / carer and reassured at lengthening intervals of 2, 4, 10 minutes and although soothed is not picked up.

For the participants of this study, sleep deprivation and concerns about establishing good sleep routines were commonly voiced at this juncture, which is in stark contrast with Mercer's (1986) study finding that only 5% of mothers complained of sleep deprivation at 4 months postpartum. Mercer estimated that approximately two thirds of interviewed mothers were having a full night's sleep at this stage (p. 170). More recent studies have shown that infant sleeping continues to be problematic for a considerable portion of mothers at 6 months and particularly so for middle-class mothers (Fisher et al., 2002; Hiscock & Wake, 2001). St James-Roberts et al. (1996) suggest that mothers of firstborn infants are particularly likely to seek help for infant crying and maternal inexperience is postulated as a causal factor. Issues of maternal infant attachment also feature prominently as predictive of sleep disturbances in the neonate, with strong maternal emotional ties to the infant associated with more night-time parenting and feeding (Scher & Dror, 2003). In contrast, McNamara, Belsky and Fearon (2003) suggested insecure infant attachment was predictive of disordered sleep patterns.

Overall, recent literature supports the premise that sleep disturbances are common in infancy, but there is additionally a growing social trend of intolerance to sleep disturbances beyond 6 months of age. Whereas a generation ago, mothers often accepted infant sleep disturbances, contemporary women, particularly economically advantaged mothers, are likely to embrace behavioural programs, such as controlled crying (Ferber, 1987, 1999) to assist in 'correcting' sleep disturbances. More traditional methods of establishing infant settling routines of bath, feed and story (Brazelton, 1992; Brazelton & Sparrow, 2001) are employed initially with behavioural programs accessed usually only when other methods fail to have the desired effect.

Although sleep schools are becoming increasingly common, as yet, they receive scant attention in research literature. However, the idea of sleep 'training' has invaded popular literature and novels such as 'Babyville' by Jane Green (2001) and parenting magazines discuss sleep training in infants. What research literature exists, suggests that these interventions effect an improvement in infant sleep patterns (Hanna & Rolls, 2001; Long, 2003; Sykes, 1999), but that the effects of the intervention may be short-lived (Hawkins-Walsh, Hiscock & Wake, 2003). In this study, sleep centres and controlled crying were last resorts for many sleep-deprived participants, who then displayed defensiveness and angst in their choices. Mothers were concerned about good sleep habits in the infant and ensuring their own health by securing sufficient sleep, similar to findings in a small body of literature. Rowe (2003), who conducted a qualitative narrative study of 21 middle-class mothers of infants, aged 1-12 months, discussed issues of "sustaining self through getting enough sleep" (p. 188). Interestingly, mothers in Rowe's study believed that neonates could or should learn to sleep for long night periods, from soon after birth (p. 187). Mothers in the current study similarly expressed dismay when at three months of age the infant still awoke frequently at night.

SIDS

Generally speaking, the worry of sudden infant death syndrome was much diminished by 4-6 months, though it was still present in some form for most, if not all, the study mothers. Again 'career women' were highly represented. Interestingly, for the women who had returned to work earlier than 6 months, SIDS was seldom listed as a concern, possibly because more pressing concerns of co-coordinating work and childcare eclipsed less immediate worries such as SIDS. However, for some women, concerns relating to SIDS continued to be significant at 6 months postpartum. For example, Rosie [career woman], a computer expert, was intimately familiar with ratios and statistical odds. For her, SIDS statistics of 1:1000 were considerably worrisome:

> *I know it's useful to say, you know, 'don't smoke and but once you've done that, you have that kind of anxiety, well, they say it's a leading cause of death in babies under one year! Can the leading cause of death be small? I think it's one out of a thousand now? Isn't it? It was 1: 500 but it's fallen to 1:1000, but 1:1000 is not small! 1:1000 is high, when you think of the vaccine, it's 1:100,000!*

In general, concerns about SIDS receive scant acknowledgement within the literature relating to motherhood experiences after 3 months. However, high rates of maternal anxiety around SIDS after 6 months of age appear to be unusual. In 1986, Mercer reported that few mothers expressed concerns about SIDS at 4 months postpartum (p. 166) and successive studies enumerating maternal concerns at this juncture fail to mention SIDS as a leading concern (Berryman & Windridge, 1995; Nelson, 2003b; Sethi, 1995; Smith, 1999; Tarkka, 2003). One possible explanation for the increased levels of concern displayed by this study's participants may relate to what Easterbrooks (1988), describes as the 'vulnerable child syndrome'. Parents experiencing anxiety around the child's vulnerability were noted to "persist in their concerns about minor …illnesses and act in an overprotective manner" (p. 182). Indeed, Ferketich and Mercer (1990), found that pregnancy risk and anxiety had long reaching consequences and continued to affect family functioning, parental competency and state anxiety at 8 months postpartum (p. 134).

158

Finally, advice on infant sleep is largely informed by the medical and public health discourses underpinning SIDS prevention campaigns (Rowe, 2003). In particular, the 'back to sleep' campaign in Australia has received considerable media coverage and the associated reduction of SIDS has led to wholesale endorsement of the movement. A plethora of research and literature has resulted (Gerard, Harris & Thach, 2002; Hunt et al., 2003; Willinger, Ko, Hoffman, Kessler & Corwin, 2003). Information-seeking quests using infant sleep as keywords yield publications focusing mostly on SIDS prevention, which possibly results in an inflated impression of the prevalence of this serious condition, common to that experienced by several participants in this study.

In the following section, issues of self for the mothers of this study are addressed.

Issues of self / wanting to keep something of myself

'Wanting to keep something of myself' continues as described in chapter 5, though at this stage of 4-6 months it takes on a new dimension, that of 'getting the mix right'. Mothers, particularly career women, discuss trying to find the right balance between work and family. There is a departure from early ideas of mothering as an adjunct to the participant's work life and a re-negotiation of self and life goals. For Cassie [career woman], achieving a balance was critical:

> *The balance is quite critical, especially when you are older, when you are younger you don't understand what balance is, it's quite important to have a balance ... I kept all my things [work and childcare] going and as much as that's hard it still maintained, you know [who I am].*

For Margaret [career woman], not relinquishing entirely to the maternal role was important:

> *Also trying to find that mix between me as a person and Harry's mother, ... I don't want to be just the mother I'll have the mix if I can.*

Among the dream-come-true mothers, this sense of balance is less clearly articulated. Some like Janet were 'happy to be able to stay-at-home' and were clearly untroubled by issues of self:

I'm more content! To be able to just stay-at-home, to just go to mother' group or to go shoppin. I don't need to be in all the shops and in all the trendy clothes and trendy shoes ... I don't need to do that, my life is my family!

Although the struggles and difficulties experienced by women, when balancing work and family, have been prodigiously attended within the literature, (Filene, 1998; Freely & Pyper, 1993; Glenn, 1994; Granrose & Kaplan, 1996; Grieve, 1986; Hattery, 2001; Hoffnung, 1995; Johnson & Johnson, 1980; Keller, 1994; Weingarten, 1994), achieving balance in respect to maternal self definition is less well addressed. Mercer (1986) discussed employment as a major concern for mothers at 4 months postpartum and more recently, Leonard (1993), in her doctoral study, examined stress and coping in first-time mothers with career commitments. Leonard discovered that mothers experienced a change in self-concept within their mothering roles. Interestingly, Leonard further found that study participants had expected mothering to "add a role to their repertoire, when, in fact, they experienced motherhood as world transforming", which then precipitated a change in life goals and a new self-understanding (viii), which is very similar to this study's findings. Smith-Pierce (1994), too, described a sense of conflict in balancing work and child and discussed a shift in maternal priorities away from work. Meanwhile, Barlow and Cairns (1997) studied mothering as a psychological experience and spoke of "engaging in the process of self-socialisation" (p. 232) and re-negotiating self. This re-negotiation of self involved a revision of priorities, particularly around work and mothering. Changing maternal priorities are further discussed in chapter 7.

What follows now is an exploration of concerns related to socialisation of the infant, particularly as it relates to the social development of the family.

Social concerns / how we will develop as a family

Concerns around social development of the infant and of the family, were again articulated more commonly, though not exclusively, among the career women. Just as with other concerns, mothers described a more expansive range of worries particularly around the optimum degree of socialisation for the infant and the development of the family unit. Margaret [career woman] explains:

I worry about how we are going to develop as a family. I hope I'm socialising him enough ... you don't want to put too much pressure on yourself as a parent too. It's hard enough to

do all this, let alone rush around to all those things [gymbaroo, swimming lessons, music].
There's going to be nothing left of you!

Gayle [career woman] worried considerably that her unbending attitude towards routine might seriously affect her daughter's development:

I suppose we were pretty rigid with things that we did with Tina and now I'm worried about the rigidity that we forced into her, for example we always made her sleep in a separate room, right from the beginning and you know, now I read all these things that say that that might not be a good thing for their development.

Whereas Petra's [career woman] concerns took on a more global aspect:

I think about what sort of world he'll have to cope with and when you see all the things that are going on at the moment, all the troubles and all that, what sort of world have we brought you into? All the problems and trouble and wars going to start out.

Lesser-achieving mothers too, expressed hopes and fears for their children's social development, though they were less likely to intellectualise about global events or perspectives and instead concentrated on family and social dynamics. Annie [dream-come-true] sums it up:

[I worry] just that he's going to grow up to a nice young man, things like that, just ordinary things!

Interestingly, this theme of concern around socialising the infant, receives scant recognition in the literature around transition to motherhood, but is occasionally addressed in sociological and feminist literature. In her founding text, Mercer (1986) presents one exception but found that only 8% of mothers expressed concerns about infant socialisation at 4 months, although this theme is considerably more prevalent in the current study. There is no indication in Mercer's work if the concern is age-related. Hays (1996), who discussed social discourses and maternal expectations, dedicated an entire chapter to 'intensive mothering' and prescribed socialisation of the infant. Her view of 'intensive mothering' discussed in chapter 2, is closely aligned with the experiences of the career women in the

161

current study. Thurer (1994) also discusses the enormous burden imposed by contemporary expectations of middle-class mothering. Attendance at ballet, gym sessions and swim sessions are often regarded as mandatory for social and psychosocial development. Notions of advanced learning and a limited window of opportunity to avail of particularly receptive periods in the infant's development have fuelled this move towards active socialisation of the infant. Older professional mothers in this study, conditioned to exacting standards of excellence and often with considerable income, seemed to wholeheartedly embrace this movement.

It's dull

Other impressions voiced by a small segment of the career women's group, were the associated tedium and dullness of stay-at-home mothering. For Harriet, used to the excitement of a busy teaching career, being at home was a dull experience:

The most exciting part of the day is having a shower in the morning!

Kerri found she needed to *"make some of the days different"*. She tended to set herself a task a day to relieve the tedium:

I give myself a task a day, like seeing you today [interview], or go up to the shops ... I still get quite frustrated with Phil [husband], which is really unfair ... like he will do anything I ask him, but he still doesn't quite understand how monotonous it is.

Abigail felt stifled by the constraints of domesticity:

I suppose there are times when I feel very burdened, not by looking after her, but by all the ancillary things you have to do, one thing I don't like is staying home doing housework.

M&CHNs also recognised the boredom associated with stay-at-home mothering for career women. Cathy explains:

Some of them are very isolated particularly if they've come from that career background, I can remember one mother, ... a career type person and ... she said to me, 'I know what I'm doing at home, it's all settled', she said 'but, gee, it's boring ... I really can't wait to get back to work ... I love my baby and everything, but this is not the sort of life I'm used to.

In contrast, women of the dream-come-true group seldom described stay-at-home mothering as dull, but were more likely to iterate like Janet, that *'this is my life now'*

In the literature, the only reference found relating to the tedium of early mothering was located in Mercer's study. Mercer found that approximately 3% of mothers in her study described feeling bored at 4 months postpartum.

Summary

In conclusion, chapter 6 has discussed maternal experience at 4-6 months postpartum, as described by the participants of this study. There was an under-lying theme of giving in and letting go, as mothers came to realise that surrendering to infant needs was a more effective way to move forward in the transition to motherhood. At this stage, a change in maternal attitude from competing to accepting is noted, and mothers now spoke of 'giving in' to the infant's needs, realising that it was simply 'not worth it' to continue as previously. Mothers now also spoke of getting to know their infants and of recognising infant cries as purposeful and as relating principally to hunger or fatigue. Infant interaction made 4-6 months postpartum a pleasant stage for most mothers and many describe seeing their infant as a 'little person' now rather than the overwhelming responsibility he/she had been until this point. Mothers also describe finding their own way as they realise that the there is no single 'right way' to care for an infant. This understanding then gave rise to an altered maternal approach and women discussed tailoring their care activities to their infant's needs and their individual circumstances. A newfound maternal confidence also facilitated maternal decision making and participants constantly referred to 'things getting better' at this juncture.

Concerns about the infant and quality of mothering were now considerably diminished and a less expansive range of concerns was reported, including principally, sleep difficulties and SIDS. The unsettled infant continued to be problematic for many mothers, particularly those mothers already returned to work. There was an emphasis on 'trying to fix the problem' of poor sleeping patterns and several career mothers discussed controlled crying and attendance at sleep schools. Younger and less accomplished mothers in this study were less likely to resort to these means to secure sleep. Maternal concerns around socialisation of the infant are also discussed here and differences are again noted between categories of participants, with the more accomplished mothers describing a more expansive range of concerns than other mothers. Maternal attempts 'to keep something of myself' and preserve some modicum of their prior lives are also considered.

In chapter 7, aging and maternal identity are analysed together with the theme 'feeling like a mother' as participants reflect on their journey to motherhood. Issues of returning to work and changing personal priorities are also reviewed. Finally, social expectations of mothering as they relate to contemporary discourses are briefly reviewed.

CHAPTER 7

FEELING LIKE A MOTHER

I only have to look at her, it's the best thing I've ever done in my life, it's the most frightening thing I've ever done in my life, you know when people say I've done a lot of silly things and I've done a lot of wrong things but this is the best thing I've ever done in my life!

Chapter 7 represents the final temporal stage in the transition to motherhood for the participants of this study. The underlying theme is that of 'feeling like a mother' and, at this stage, mothers described 'really enjoying' their mothering experiences. By six months postpartum the mood was overwhelming positive and accounts were sprinkled with claims of satisfaction, such as 'it's the best thing I've ever done'. Much emphasis was placed on the simplicity and purity of loving and being loved by an infant. Mothers spoke of feeling awed and overwhelmed to find themselves the recipients of the infant's 'unconditional love'. There was a departure from earlier ideas of mothering as an adjunct to the participants' lives and instead women described a newfound understanding of 'what was important' in their lives. A re-organisation of maternal priorities was evident at this stage, together with a re-negotiation of self and life goals. In general, this redefinition of maternal philosophy was devoid of the 'self' struggles that marked early motherhood.

Most study participants discussed concerns about the aging body and indeed, many of the women's stories were prefaced with 'as an older mother'. It soon became obvious that age was important in the mother's newly acquired maternal self and a clear phase of re-framing past life history was noted as mothers appraised their circumstances, redefined and reinvented themselves, not merely as women or mothers, but as older mothers. Comparisons to younger mothers were common, as were references to increasing life expectancies and better health and longevity, contemporarily. Throughout, there was a sense that their advanced maturity and more settled lifestyle had contributed positively to their satisfaction with and their greater adaptation to the maternal role. There was additionally an oft-expressed suggestion of having 'been there, done that' and of having no unfinished business. Women thus felt ready to move forward in life and to mother. Principal concerns centred around returning to work and balancing work and family while retaining sufficient energy to 'be there' for the child.

In this chapter, several factors are discussed as impacting significantly on the experience of maternity for older first-time mothers. Firstly, maternal age as a component of mothering identity is addressed, followed by an exploration of the theme 'feeling like a mother'. The following section addresses maternal employment, principally returning to work and balancing work and family. Next, a discussion of changing maternal philosophies and priorities is attended as women come to evaluate what is important and to make choices in their lives. Then social implications of later timing of pregnancy are discussed, together with maternal experiences of the social mores surrounding new mothering.

Age and the maternal self

Throughout the data analysis of this study a recurrent presenting thread was that of older maternal age which is one of the study's five main themes. This theme was expressed differently at various junctures of the pregnant and new mother's life, as related to risk perception during pregnancy, to perceptions of heightened infant vulnerability in the perinatal and neonatal periods, and finally, in terms of maternal health and mortality as the mothers achieved transition to motherhood. Most mothers had, by this stage, incorporated age into their maternal selves and had built a picture of themselves as older mothers. There were three mothers in this study who considered age to be unimportant and felt instead that maternal 'personality' was the important key to successful maternal adaptation. For the majority, maternal age was clearly important and at 6 months postpartum most mothers continued to explore what age meant in their lives. Comparisons to younger mothers were common, as were examples illustrating how much better participants were suited to maternity at this juncture, compared to an earlier age. References to increasing life expectancies and better health contemporarily, extending deep into old age, also presented. Throughout, mothers appraised their circumstances, redefined and reinvented themselves, not simply as women or mothers, but as older mothers. Similar to that discussed in chapter 3, women in this study, achieved both "self-coherence and diversity" within their narratives (Holstein & Gubrium, 2000, p. 107), as they shaped and reshaped their understandings of mothering in general, and older mothering in particular. These stories allowed affirmation of the 'new' self, as in the manner suggested by Gergen (2001) as "self-identification, self-justification, self- criticism and social solidification" (p. 249).

In the current study, many age-related themes and sub-themes presented. One recurring theme was, for want of a more elegant phrase, 'been there, done that' and the women expressed few regrets in moving on with their lives. Another theme related to feeling that maternal maturity advantaged both mother and baby. Women described 'knowing myself better' as predictive of greater satisfaction with the mothering role. Concerns centred on having enough energy to 'be there' for the infant and issues related to mortality, morbidity and financial provision for the child.

'Been there, done that'

For the majority of the older participants, irrespective of career investment, there was a sense of readiness around having a child in their lives. Satisfaction with past life events such as travel and social opportunities allowed the woman to move forward and many women articulated a sense of having 'been there, done that' and of being ready for a change. For Sue [career woman], being at home and raising children was what she wanted to do with this stage of her life:

> *I think the fact that we are older means that ... both of us have done everything that we ever wanted to do! We've travelled, we're much more settled, our expectations were that we would be at home and we quite honestly don't want to do anything else.*

Participants frequently described moving away from social events such as parties and nightclubs and anticipating a more settled or family-orientated lifestyle. This was accompanied by a feeling of not missing out socially, and this trend was described by older mothers, irrespective of career investment. Adapting to lifestyle changes was not the cause for concern it might have been earlier. Petra [career woman] explains:

> *It's more that I was a lot quicker to come to terms with the changes. I think it would've been a lot harder if I were younger, like giving up things that I still hadn't finished doing yet. I think that would've been the biggest thing!*

Janet [dream-come-true]:
> *I suppose in your twenties you'd be doing other things, quite often it's the night life part of things that you enjoy most, I think I was ready for the responsibility.*

However, for some women plans to create space for childbearing and raising, fell short of their mark. Margaret [career woman] had spent several years postponing childbearing in pursuit of career and felt well prepared for family life. Nonetheless, her experiences as a new mother were not as anticipated.

167

We sort of thought we were past a lot of things that we weren't going to miss, like we didn't want to go out to pubs or that. We'd done enough of that in the past so we thought we were all right, but we didn't realise we liked a lot of time to relax and read the paper and things like that. That's all gone now, I didn't realise it.

Dobrzykowski (1998) coined the term "no unfinished business" to represent a mother's satisfaction with past life events, allowing her to move on to new experiences without regret (p. 2). In her doctoral study, Dobrzykowski's found that primiparae aged over 30 who considered themselves to have no 'unfinished business' were able to move forward with their lives, whilst those women who considered they had unfinished tasks were less

well able to deal with the issues of new maternity. In this study, this notion of no 'unfinished business' emerges frequently in the accounts of career women and participants described feeling ready to move on in their lives, having completed travel and career plans. Among the lesser achieving women a considerably muted sense of this theme was found. More modest goals, such as completing landscaping and home improvements before the baby was born, were discussed. For the young achievers group, there was a sense of life continuing much as before, albeit with an interruption to plans. These young women, the majority of whom had had an unexpected pregnancy, drew on other role models who had successfully resumed career plans after childbearing. Melanie [young achiever] explains:

I definitely am sacrificing my career a bit for now ... but I look and see lots of women pick it back up again... like my obstetrician ... she had 10 years off, she's terrific and she had 10 years off.

Maternal maturity advantages both mother and baby

Various adult development theories suggest that middle adulthood is a time of crisis (Erikson, 1978, Levinson, 1996) and studies exploring women's development across the life span report that between ages 30-45, approximately 75% of women undergo a major life re-orientation (Harris, Ellicott & Holmes, 1986; Wrightsman, 1988). Levinson (1996), also suggests that women aged 33-40 are engaged in "culminating life structures" that mark the end of early adulthood and the beginning of middle adulthood (p. 334). As women aged 35-48, the participants of this study might then be expected to be at a critical stage, though little evidence of life crisis presented in their accounts. Identity issues here seemed to relate less to personal satisfaction with life achievements, than to mothering identity. There was a general sense of feeling more self-assured with advanced maternal age and participants believed they were considerably advantaged by their self-confidence and competence. This trend was most marked among career women. Abigail [career woman] explains her feelings of confidence:

I already feel far more competent than a lot of women that are 10 years younger than me! More confident, I don't feel like I'm giving up anything!

Petra [career woman] describes enjoying mothering, rather that just coping, as an advantage of greater maternal age:

I've sort of been thinking about it and I mean if I had Blake like 10 years or something earlier, ... I suppose I would've coped but I think it would've been an entirely different situation and I don't think I would've enjoyed it as much.

Knowing myself better

'Knowing myself' was frequently expressed as feeling 'comfortable about who I am' and about choices made. There was a sense of knowing 'where you are going' and although most participants acknowledged that change was part of life's continuum, there was an expectation that major changes were less likely during this life stage. A recognition that life 'wasn't perfect' is attributed to greater life experience and understanding. Kristen [career woman], explains:

I think you know who you are ... you're not going to be as perturbed by things.

For Petra, [career woman] greater self-knowledge was associated with clearer destination and goals:

And I think you know yourself a bit more' [as an older mother]. I think that makes it a bit different, knowing ... I mean, you still know there's changes to come in life and that, but you know where you're going, most of the time, at a younger age I think you are still trying to work out who you are, what's important and you've sort of been through that now.

There was a sense of understanding that life was unpredictable and many women felt that the understanding they had gained during life experiences, contributed to more tolerant and moderate attitudes. There was a tendency among the participants to describe being less 'bothered about things' and feeling they had little to prove. Harriet [career woman] explains:

An advantage of being an older mother in that I can say quite comfortably and confidently, 'no, you can't do it all'.

This sense of not being perturbed by the 'little things' is in stark contrast to earlier uncertainties and worries expressed by the women and reflects a temporal move along the transition continuum. In an earlier interview Kerri [career woman] was clearly perturbed by lack of predictability in her life as a new mother and expressed frustration with her inability to plan ahead or make appointments. Now, Kerri describes feeling unperturbed by life's little hiccups:

I think I just let things bounce off me whereas I think I would have taken them in at a younger age. I think oh well, who cares?

Others, like Kerri, when reminded of earlier concerns, happily acknowledged their initial disquiet but had 'moved on'. Despite popular opinion of mothers over 35 years, as disadvantaged by being older, participants here seldom shared that view. For many, there was a sense of having chosen a particularly appropriate time to have a baby. Petra [career woman], felt she had chosen the best time possible:

I think, I mean, I think I've chosen the best time personally the best time to do it!

Kerri [career woman] described having the time now to do justice to mothering, whereas earlier in her career, she wouldn't have had the time to devote to an infant:

I mean, at an earlier age I just wouldn't have done a baby any justice at all, I just wouldn't have had the time.

Feeling less self-orientated was also viewed as a positive experience, as Jeanne [dream-come-true], describes:

170

The good things, probably not worrying so much about your self, not caring so much about me, me, me sort of thing, you learn to be a bit selfless, your baby, so that was good!

For Margaret [career woman], a serendipitous finding was not taking herself so seriously:

I probably took myself seriously in my job and now, you can't take yourself seriously when you've got a baby.

Age-related concerns

Age-related concerns were often expressed by participants and related principally to having enough energy to keep up with the infant and to 'be there' for him/her. Many mothers discussed having considerably more energy when younger and worried about coping with a teenager when in their fifties / sixties. However, for the most part these concerns were balanced by an understanding that individuals live longer, healthier lives contemporarily and several women considered that an infant / young child would 'keep them young'. Other concerns centred around maternal health and mortality. Here Kristen [career woman] described having more energy as a younger woman:

I think if you're younger, like a lot lot younger, like in your twenties, you probably have a lot more patience, energy.

Jennifer [dream-come-true] felt similarly:

I was surprised [at] the energy levels ... you just don't [have the energy] ... in your twenties you could go all night ... go to a party and go to work the next day and think I feel fine or whatever!

Anthea [career woman] viewed the difference in fatigue as an older or younger mother as simply relative and felt other life circumstances and satisfaction with her life to date balanced the negative effects of advanced maternal age:

I'll tell you what I really thought, things like getting older and not as physically fit, that'll be harder, I honestly don't think it made a big difference! I'm tired anyway, I wake up

171

every morning and say I'm tired, you'd come home at the end of the day and say I'm tired,
I don't know how much different it would be if I was 25, probably I would've had a bit
more energy, but maybe I feel I would have resented, no not resented, ... disappointed that
I couldn't do some of the things. There really isn't that disappointment, I was ready for it.
You're probably a bit more set up by then and we're not stressing about money all the time.

Abigail [career woman] worried about being in her fifties with teenage children, but nonetheless felt that having young children would keep her and her partner young:

I suppose, I suppose Greg and I are concerned that we are going to be in our 50s looking
after teenagers when I really don't want or feel like running after an irascible 14 year old,
like I'm really going to be interested in that! But I also think it'll keep us young at heart.

Maternal health and mortality
Several mothers expressed concerns about 'being there' for the child, from a health perspective, and this was addressed by making material plans for the children in the event of their ill-health or death. Jennifer, [dream-come-true], worried a great deal about her infant being affected by parental ill-health:

And that's a concern, making sure we are around for her, you know, health-wise, that sort
of stuff.

Karine [dream-come-true] had started a bank fund for her twin boys as a safeguard against future parental ill health or demise. Death of a mother of young children known to her served as a reminder of her own mortality:

Their great-grandmother has already sent them a bit of money   So I want to start
bankbooks for them straight away ... I worry that I won't be around I think that's my
biggest concern, I was hoping at least to make it to their twentieth birthday ... like when
they're 30 I'll be 70 and hopefully I will reach 70 ... I think that ... to be there for them,
into an older age and to see them grow up ... that's my one worry, to make sure I'm around
long enough for them to be taken care of.

172

Although this aspect of maternal concern around mortality is not abundantly addressed in the literature relating to mothering over 35, some references were found. Dobrzykowski and Stern (2003) found that participants in their study discussed the "overwhelming need to think about the future and the need to ensure that their child would be adequately cared for in the event of their death" (p. 246). Smith-Pierce (1994) in her heuristic study of first-time mid-life mothers also found that women often reported "a sense of their own mortality and aging" (p. vii). In both these studies participants made efforts to provide for their children in the event of their early demise, which is similar to this study's findings. At this stage a new concern came to light, relating to the social context of older mothering, which interestingly, was expressed exclusively by the dream-come-true mothers. These women worried that their children might be teased about, or ashamed of, their older parents. Jennifer [dream-come-true] explains:

I worry about being an older Mum, I worry a lot, I worry how Chloe will deal with an older mum ... I know it sounds stupid but I want to be trendy, I want to be up there. I was thinking the other day, I'd hate it if she was teased at school 'oh your Mum's old'.

Karine [dream-come-true] also expresses her concerns:

The other thing is, there is such a thing as what's socially acceptable so as these boys get older. I can't very well, for their sakes, go around looking like a frump, I don't want them to be teased or embarrassed, I hope that they'd be able to talk to me about things like that.

Berryman et al. (1999) discussed a parallel though divergent finding in her study of mothers over 35. She found that participants described being mistaken for their infant's grandmother, but in general, found it amusing rather than distressing. In contrast dream-come-true mothers here anticipated distress at being considered 'an old mother'. In this study, greater maternal confidence and self assurance seemed to have a cushioning effect and the more accomplished mothers seemed little concerned at six months, by negative social implications of aging. This finding is similar to that expressed by Dobrzykowski and Stern (2003). They found that the more confident a mother "felt about her abilities to mother successfully, the less influence the social structure had on her" (p. 248). Indeed, within the literature, there is a clear indication that greater maternal self-assurance augurs well for maternal adaptation, and successive authors have found with this theme. Feldman and Nash (1986) suggested

173

that women endowed with "ego strength and maturity become more effective mothers in a variety of situations" and also that for women, maturity, "positively predicts positive parenting" (p. 219). Belsky, Ward and Rovine (1986) also found that the personal resourcefulness of an adult was predictive of parental adaptation and functioning and Gottesman (1992) found high levels of competency among older mothers. Indeed, a host of studies underscored greater maternal age and maturity as predictive of greater maternal adaptation and satisfaction in the mothering role (Berryman, 1991, Berryman et al., 1999; Pridham & Chang, 1992; Ragozin et al., 1982). At this juncture, the majority of older participants reported feeling largely immune to negative social discourses, though some, admittedly a small percentage, felt these discourses to be destructive to the new mother's confidence and adaptation. Abigail [career woman] explains:

> *The over emphasis on the problems that older women have is very destructive and I really*
> *want to emphasise that point ... to her capacity to just roll into the roll.*

Issues of self and sustaining self, as distinct from but linked to maternal age, were frequently voiced by the participants of this study and are addressed in the following section.

Issues of self

Similar to that discussed in chapters 5 and 6, issues of self and sustaining self were raised throughout this study, though, at this point, it was with decreasing angst and urgency. Whereas in the earlier interviews, there was a tendency towards self-abnegation in favour of perceived infant needs, now the mood veers towards compromise. The theme 'finding my own way' presents here as a growing understanding that 'mothers have needs too'. Most participants described reaching a stage of allowing themselves occasional 'time off', understanding that to do so did not make them derelict in their duty to the infant. Once again, issues of self were most commonly raised by career women and to a lesser extent by young achievers. Dream-come-true mothers, in general, did not address issues of 'sustaining self' in this study, but were more likely to claim 'this is my life now'. Sustaining self manifested as needing a break occasionally from the infant and understanding that mothers too had needs.

Doing something for myself / needing a break

Several mothers, again primarily career women, described needing a break from the intensity and constancy of mothering and, by six months, had redefined the role sufficiently to take some time off, on occasion. This time off was generally described as 'doing something for myself'. Petra [career woman] explains:

> *I did an embroidery course that was ... it was two weeks, a Saturday and then another Saturday five weeks later because you had to get all your stuff done and then bring it back ... and just that day to yourself was very very nice [Laughter] ... it was good and people saying 'well, did you miss him'? No! [Laughter] he was fine and his Dad had a great time.*

For some mothers, however, describing a 'need' for time off was difficult. Anthea's [career woman] account of taking time off to go to the movies is tinged with defensiveness:

> *There are times when I'll go off, I'll just sneak off to the movies by myself and Eric will mind him, just to have a break ... well, I need it, when you think you've had 35 years of your life doing what you want, when you want, how you want and then all of a sudden I can't do all those things because I've got him.*

Meanwhile Gayle [career woman] reassured herself that her having time out allowed the father-infant bond to develop:

> *My only break from her now, apart from work, which I consider a break is when I go to my piano lesson and Mark looks after her on Wednesday night, and he has some time with her...*

At this stage, although the infant's needs continued to be paramount, mothers understood infant crying as no longer constituting the urgency of earlier days and, whenever possible, mothers also made efforts to accommodate their own needs.

My needs are important too

This recognition of maternal needs as important marks a departure from earlier days of mothering, when the new mother often felt unable to shower or dress until her partner returned from work to take over care of the infant. Karine [dream-come-true] discusses meeting her basis needs:

175

I think one of the things they said in hospital was that my needs came first, because if my needs weren't met then I couldn't efficiently meet their needs. My needs are having a shower, going to the toilet and just having, shoving in a piece of toast, I mean, it was like that!

Other issues of self include personal reflection, renegotiation of self and life goals and feeling like a creditable woman.

Personal reflection / re-negotiation of self and life goals

From a life span perspective, midlife is often described as a time of taking stock of one's life to date (Erikson, 1978; Levinson, 1996) and of re-evaluating life goals and self, before moving forward. In this study, a re-negotiation of self and life goals was evident among all the older participants, irrespective of career accomplishment, though once again, the more accomplished women were more likely to philosophise and intellectualise about their experiences. Harriet [career woman] describes pausing to reflect:

It's been personally, a really good way to take time out from my career to be able to have an excuse to reflect, to reflect on what I think is important and to look within myself at my value system.

At this stage there was a marked departure from earlier ideas of mothering as an adjunct to the participants' lives and a newfound understanding of 'what is important'. A re-organisation of maternal priorities was evident and, in general, this redefinition of maternal philosophy was devoid of the 'self' struggles that marked early motherhood. For Angela, [dream-come-true] pride in her home often ruled her decisions around activities in the earlier days of mothering. Now she describes feeling that her daughter is 'more important':

She's more important, whereas I used to be really very proud of my house ... it's not important any more, I don't care if I've got toys rolling around, I don't care if I can't get the ironing done until the morning, it doesn't really matter...

For Laura [career woman] re-evaluating and changing life philosophies allowed her to view her daughter as the most important element of her life:

> *I think the best thing is actually just Emily and seeing her smile or watching her sleep, anything really at the end of the day, it's really all that's important! That's a big change from 2 years ago, I suppose then I would have said it was still my family, but my job would've come really close! ... But now, I don't know that it runs a close second even though I give it a lot of me!*

Becoming a creditable woman

The notion of achieving full womanhood in becoming a mother was voiced by a small but persistent percentage of participants, though the tendency showed no marked preference for any one group. For Rosie [career woman] coming from a culture that placed considerable emphasis on the mothering role, having a baby was seen as establishing her credibility as a bona fide woman:

> *I'm now a creditable woman, so that's a kind of change!*

For Jennifer, [dream-come-true], whose previous life, by her own admission, lacked definition, having a baby represented taking on an 'adult' and responsible role:

> *I guess it sounds silly at my age and stage but I think a lot of women think 'my God it's a grown up thing to do', when you haven't had a baby it's such a mature thing to do! It's the responsible thing to do, Gosh!*

Although this notion of 'motherhood proving womanhood' is not abundantly reported among the mothers of this study, it remains an established concept within the literature, contested principally by feminist debates. Indeed, when searching for literature relating to this theme I was surprised to note how frequently the notion of mothering and becoming a woman were co-associated, for example, in the following book titles: Bergum, V. (1997). A child on her mind: the experience of becoming a woman, Bergum, V. (1989). Woman to mother: a transformation, Brown et al. (1994), Missing Voices: the experience of womanhood, discussing postnatal depression and morbidity and Kitzinger, S. (1980) Women as mothers. Within the transition to motherhood literature, Mercer (1986) found that many women described childbearing as a " transition to adulthood and admission to a new social status" (p. 319) and Leifer (1980) discussed numerous instances of women associating pregnancy and childbearing with achieving full womanhood (pp. 161-167). Historical tomes are replete with traditional notions of mothering as essential to full womanly status. For example, Grayzel (1997), studied mothering roles around WWI and suggests that mothering came to "represent for women what soldiering did for men", a "gender-specific" and important role (p. 122). After WWII, Dally (1982), described an era of idealisation of motherhood (p. 92), with the mothering role central to full womanly status. As discussed in chapter 2, feminist critiques from the 1950s/1960s, however, are dismissive of the notion of mothering = womanhood, regarding it as patriarchal (De Beauvoir, 1952; Eisenstein, 1984; Friedan, 1963; Greer, 1970). More recently, from the 1980s, there is a clear change of mood, following the introduction of the notion of choice into childbearing. One possible explanation for the low numbers of mothers recounting this notion in the current study, may rest in the fact that most mothers were highly accomplished in other fields and thus may not have felt the necessity of mothering from a personal development point of view. An alternate view may be that in contemporary advanced and cosmopolitan post-industrial societies, such as that in Melbourne, traditional notions of mothering as essential to womanhood may not hold much sway.

Discussion

Chronological age is often used as a marker for social maturity (Baltes, 1987) and personal maturity, related to chronological age, is often suggested as a predictor of maternal adjustment (Belsky et al., 1986; Feldman & Nash, 1986; Gottesman, 1992). However, few studies of maternal adjustment have featured age-related comparisons. Of the studies surveyed, a variety of opinions have emerged. Most evidence suggests that advanced maternal age, higher levels of education and primiparity are associated with poorer social support and higher expectations of self, all of which foreshadow poorer maternal adjustment. Paradoxically, the available studies relating to maternal adjustment among older mothers do not support this premise. Rossi (1980) suggests that being 'out of time' socially for such life events as marriage and childbearing, results in decreased social re-enforcement and may "trigger anxiety because the individual's cultural expectation of appropriate timing has been violated" (p. 12). Dobrzykowski and Stern (2003) found that their participants, later-timing American mothers, all spoke of "being out of sync" with mainstream American views of when a woman should become a mother (p. 248), although this feeling was only voiced by one of the 'dream-come-true mothers' in the current study. One possible explanation for this finding is the lower median age for childbearing in the U.S.A.

and the relatively lower, though increasing, rate of primigravidae over 35. In Australia, age over 35 is more commonly seen among primigravid women, which may contribute to greater acceptance and normalisation.

In Mercer's (1986) seminal study, there was a suggestion that older and more educated mothers had higher expectations of self and fared less well than younger mothers, particularly in the early days of mothering. Belsky et al. (1986) also identified maternal age and education as factors significantly impacting on maternal adjustment and Pridham, Lytton, Chang and Rutledge (1991), who conducted a study into the early postpartum transition of American mothers (n = 108), found that higher levels of education contributed negatively to maternal adjustment. Psychologist Myra Leifer's (1980) study, reviewing the experiences of 19, mostly tertiary-educated, primigravid white women aged 22-33, found that "among the more educated women ... worry about the ability to be a good mother was even more pronounced" (p. 157). Finally, Falk (2000) observed that the well-educated mothers, aged over 28, interviewed in her doctoral study, experienced conflict between the needs of mother and baby and further interpreted the women's defensiveness as related to pressure to "conform to cultural representations and social expectations associated with motherhood" (p. v).

In general, social support is portrayed as lacking for the older primipara (Ambler Walter, 1986; Mercer, 1986; Reece, 1995; Rubin, 1967b) and a host of studies have underscored support as an important mediator for subsequent maternal adjustment (Barclay et al., 1997; Dennis et al., 2002; Fleming et al., 1988; Reece, 1995; Tarkka, 2003; Tarkka & Paunonen, 1996). Indeed, older primiparity has traditionally been associated with maternal maladjustment. This association however, is not well supported in much of the literature dealing with the experiences of older primigravidae, such as: Berryman and Windridge (1995); Feldman and Nash (1986); Gottesman (1992); Grossman, Eichler and Winickoff (1980); Lederman (1984); Ragozin et al. (1982). Indeed, more nurturing behaviour and more optimal interaction with the infant has frequently been linked to increased maternal age (Feldman & Nash, 1986; Gottesman, 1992; Grossman et al., 1980). Green and Kafetsios (1997) who conducted a large prospective study of new mothers aged 21-35 mothers at approximately 6 weeks postpartum, (n = 1285), found that the data did not support the "stereotypical notion that women with high expectations are setting themselves up for failure and disappointment" (p. 155).

Indeed, a number of studies suggest that older maternal age is associated with greater satisfaction with parenting (Berryman et al., 1999; Berryman & Windridge, 1995; Ragozin et al., 1982) and greater commitment to the role (Berryman 1991; Ragozin et al., 1982). There is also some suggestion that "social advantage may make up for biological disadvantage" for the children of older mothers (Stein &

179

Susser, 2000, p. 1681). Stein and Susser also conclude that improvements in economic measures among older parents influence better performance at school among their offspring. This finding of better performance at school and on cognitive testing is echoed in other studies, for example: Gross, Mettelman, Dye and Slagle (2001); Heck, Schoendorf, Ventura and Kiely (1997); Pollock (1996) and Zybert, Stein and Belmont (1978). There is additionally a suggestion within the literature that older mothers are more likely to feel accomplished and self-fulfilled and therefore less likely to expect their children to contribute to their sense of fulfilment (Berryman, 1991).

In her comparative study, Gottesman (1992) went one step further to suggest that older maternal age might actually be advantageous to maternal adaptation. She found that younger women experienced more difficulty in prenatal adjustment to the maternal role, than did middle (25-29) and later (over 30) child-bearers, displaying a more 'bothered' attitude about changes in appearance related to pregnancy. Windridge and Berryman (1996) concurred with this finding, indicating that older mothers were less likely to be concerned about body image than younger women. In the current study, mothers generally felt that age and maturity equipped them well for their maternal experiences and considered that they had greater reserves of patience than perhaps at a younger age. In the following section, achieving the transition to motherhood is addressed.

Feeling like a mother / achieving the transition

> *Sometimes it takes a while to think ' I'm a mother!' ... It's a big role and I think it takes a while to [assimilate it], being a mother isn't changing nappies and things, that's just a practical thing! Basically as they develop it's the emotional and working out what he's thinking and how he feels is an entirely different ball game than just being a cow. So that's when I think you actually become a mother... in tune with them, and he looks at you and goes 'what's going on?' and wants a cuddle and all those sorts of things ... that's when your mother role comes in, that's when you feel it, bonding in a different way though and you become a mother.*

Whereas mothers of the 'dream-come-true' group were at odds to understand the question 'when did you start to feel like a mother? And generally described feeling like a mother once the infant was born, career women and young achievers described assimilating or 'working into the role'. For these women, six months postpartum seemed to be a particular marker and most described 'feeling like a mother' after this time. Many were self-congratulatory at having 'made it' thus far. There was a general

180

understanding of the magnitude of the maternal role and a changing appreciation of what it meant to be a mother. Most participants made a clear distinction between the care activities of early mothering associated with getting through each day and later feelings of being 'bonded' with, and proud of, their infants. For Kelly [career woman], there was a real sense of pride in herself for having achieved such a strong bond with her infant, as her humorous account illustrates:

And you know when the bond thing just kicks in ... Awww I felt so proud of myself, the bond was so strong and you'd do anything ... killing this big hunk for threatening my baby ... superwoman da da [laughter].

For Jane [career woman], feeling really 'proud' of her son helped diminish her initial anxieties and balance the overwhelming responsibility of the role:

It's a big responsibility but at least it doesn't scare me as much as it did initially ... I think there's another part of me that's so proud of him and happy with him and it's like, you know, so this is what it's like to be a mother, oh it's a brilliant feeling and its not all scary!

Whereas for Janet [dream-come-true], the maternal role was easily and immediately assimilated:
I felt almost instantly and almost every day it expounds [sic] it, that it is a role I was always meant to play.

In addition to being at odds to understand the question 'when did you start to feel like a mother?' dream-come-true mothers tended to veer away from questions of this nature, dismissing them as impractical and inconsequential. Janet explains:

I can't be doing with all this motherhood stuff.

For Janet, mothering was a normal part of everyday life, rather than an exceptional event requiring education and preparation. Although the majority of participants had reached a stage of 'feeling like a mother' by six months postpartum, it was not an exclusive achievement. Women whose pregnancies had been particularly anxiety provoking and who had effectively distanced themselves from perceivably vulnerable pregnancies, appeared to have a slower than usual assimilation of maternal identity. Karine [dream-come-true], whose twin pregnancy had been particularly terrifying, spent several weeks on bed rest fearing the worst, before her infants were born safely at term. Six months later she described not yet having 'made the connection':

I guess I still don't feel like I'm a mother ... I mean I know I'm a Mum but I guess I haven't made that connection yet.

Kerri [career woman] had had her baby because she recognised that she was running out of time. However, feeling like a mother, or indeed remembering that she was a mother, seemed difficult:

Sometimes I catch myself saying 'Aunty Kristy' and have to say 'no, Mum'.

Enjoying it more / my wonderful baby
For the majority of participants, the mood was overwhelmingly positive at six months postpartum. Women spoke of the purity and simplicity of an infant's love in a complicated world and particularly valued the joy and pleasure of 'tiny things'. Most were amazed at their unanticipated depth of feeling towards the infant and the reciprocal and unconditional love of that infant. Margaret explains:

I think it's very pure, the joy of it is very pure, but the downside is very pure too [laughter] ... just so much in life is complicated and you have to work through you know, just how we entertain ourselves and we go out to dinner and babies, it's just pure and he can give us such joy with the tiniest things.

For Jennifer [dream-come-true], the pleasure of her infant's unconditional love and faith in her mother, got her through the not-so-pleasant times:

Yeah, I'll be driving along in the car and she'll be in the back, like the other day, she was killing herself laughing and it was just that ... 'little friend' ... a real little friend! That just accepts you, she looks at you with such loving and that sort of thing, she has such faith in you, ... in one way it tears you apart and you want to be perfect for her, but in another way it gives you great joy, great joy that she loves you so much and unconditionally and they bring you such fun, ... I mean 90% is not fun but that little bit keeps you going!

Many mothers described a sense of being 'rewarded everyday with something he/she does' and indeed several [principally career women] became emotional when discussing how they had almost missed out on the experience of childbearing, during years of procrastination and prevarication. Several described feeling different now as a woman and unanimously discussed their limited prior understanding of 'what it was to be a mother'. In general, the new and unanticipated dimension mothering brought to their lives far exceeded expectations. Jane [career woman] explains:

Its amazing that sense of and I suppose everyone has it ... but I've never experienced it in all my life, sometimes I'll just be sitting there, ... and he'll be on my knee and he'll look up at me and smile ... it's like this wave ... my breath sort of goes, its like this amazing strong sense of love, ... you know I spent most of my life being very happy, having a great family and loving my family and my partner, but its an extraordinary feeling ... I think you look at him and when he looks at you ... you think about how much, how unconditional his love is and you sort of think ... it makes you feel pretty special.

Although not abundantly addressed within the literature, this suggestion of unanticipated depth of feeling for the infant is found in studies of older mothering. Crittenden (2001) found that highly accomplished corporate mothers had not anticipated the "degree to which they would fall in love with their new baby" (p. 34) and Smith-Pierce (1994) found that mothers reported an unexpected depth of love for the child. Cudmore (1997) who examined the experiences of 6 primiparae aged 28-36, also found that women reported an unanticipated intensity of bond with the child. Mothers in this study frequently made reference to feeling blessed with a particularly 'good' or easy baby, which seems to be in keeping with growing maternal appreciation and love.

Recommend it highly

In general, mothers in this study said they would highly recommend mothering and several spoke of urging friends and sisters to avail of reducing opportunities to mother. Most affirmed that this was a life experience 'not to be missed'. Margaret [career woman] describes her new understanding of being a mother and her concerns that her sisters shouldn't 'miss out':

Oh I just didn't realise what was involved, how much different it is as a woman, being a mother and if you don't do it you're missing out ...

I've got 2 older sisters that haven't had children and I just want to say to them, do it, do it now! Just risk it!

For some, notably three of the career women, theirs was not an unequivocal recommendation. Rather, it was tinged with an urgency to understand the burdens of social expectations around mothering and the life-changing qualities of childbearing. Interestingly, among even the dissenting voices, there was an understanding of burdensome social mores rather than burdensome mothering. Kerri [career woman] describes the advice she gives to a friend over 35 contemplating childbearing:

I didn't take the decision lightly, but it's so different to what I thought, I say to her 'think about it, if you're not sure' ... it is a huge financial change and if she talks about going back to work after ... and I say aww! That'd break your heart, like you probably won't want to once ... I just think she will just find it so hard to work her job, which is really demanding and have a baby and go to work every day!

Cassie [career woman] states:

I think it's got to be something you really want! And it's got to be a mutual thing with your partner, because if you just want it and your partner doesn't which comes with it when you're both older. When you're older you're not as adjustable unless you want and equally, once you say we want one then, to make to try to make your life a little better and try to maintain some sort of balance to it.

In this study, older mothers in general, regardless of career commitment, found an unanticipated pleasure in their mothering experiences, similar to findings described by Berryman et al. (1999), Berryman and Windridge (1995) and Ragozin et al. (1982). In association with the unexpected depth of love most mothers felt towards their infants, maternal separation anxiety was equally unanticipated by many of the more accomplished mothers.

184

Maternal separation anxiety

This theme of maternal separation anxiety was seldom raised by young achievers and indeed did not present a dilemma for the majority of the 'dream-come-true' mothers, who tended to mother full-time. However, for the career women it proved to be an unanticipated source of angst. Expected difficulties centred on organising childcare, 'fitting it all in' and even infant separation anxiety. Few however, had considered that they would miss the infant and fret when separated from him/her. For Cassie, the strain of leaving her son and returning to work at 3 months postpartum was balanced by her rationale that she was sharing her son with other family members. Here, she explains how she never worked too far from home and frequently phoned to check that her son was 'managing'. Her angst at 'sharing her baby' is obvious:

> *The more I was generous with him it came back to me because people cared about him and I kind of feel 'you push them out early and they respond to other people' and then they're not totally dependent on you ... and I think that would have to be the key in survival! Although you really want to keep him to yourself, it's the absolute natural thing, it is hard, I suppose what went through my mind is that you never leave him that he's going to be distressed with them, ... I was never gone, especially early on, I was never gone that far away ... Being generous actually pays off but it's hard to do! Look I miss him, when I go out and I ring in to see if he's all right and I come back [to check]. That's just being a mother I think, Rick [father] doesn't do that, he doesn't ring in, but I ring ... I kind of share him more, I think, I go out to work and as much as I miss him and I like to come home and see if he is alright, it takes a lot to actually share your little boy, your little baby.*

At this stage, mothers described missing the baby when apart from him/her as distinct from merely worrying about the infant in the early days of mothering. Now the infant's company was described as 'fun' or pleasurable. For Kerri [career woman], this feeling was new and quite different from early mothering concerns:

> *In the beginning when you're not with her you'll miss her in that you're worried that she'll cry, but these days if you're gone you miss her because you just miss talking to her.*

185

Importance of family support

In general, ease of transition to motherhood was mediated by good family support. Women who considered themselves well supported and encouraged, found the transition to motherhood less onerous than others who considered themselves less well supported.

For example, Petra's mother was particularly helpful and looked after Blake while Petra [career woman] worked. It was a situation that suited everyone and Petra felt it would have been extremely difficult to manage without her family's support:

> *Sometimes I get Mum over and it gives her time with us! ... She enjoys that! ... I don't know*
> *how anyone would cope doing it by themselves and I really admire them for doing that, it's*
> *so hard. It's hard with the support, let alone by yourself!*

By six months postpartum, most mothers had managed to accommodate their circumstances and certainly career women had, by this stage, identified themselves as confident and 'street smart' in terms of accessing information and services. Nonetheless, having family support was frequently discussed as an important mediator in achieving transition. This finding sits well with established knowledge and indeed, as mentioned in chapter 5, maternal support, from a variety of sources, is well recognised within the literature as an important factor in maternal adjustment (Barclay et al., 1997; Fleming et al., 1988; Green & Kafetsios, 1997; PROBIT study group, 2001; Reece, 1995; Tarkka, 2003; Tarkka & Paunonen, 1996). Many of the study participants, especially career women, lived some distance from or were otherwise removed from their own mothers. Others had elderly or frail parents. Recourse to paid help eased the burden for these women somewhat and an unexpected source of support presented in the form of the 'new mothers' groups' run by the M&CH centres (Carolan, in press-b).

New mothers' groups

In this study, new mothers' groups were accorded immense importance by older mothers. These groups functioned as a source of access to other new parents, as a valuable reference group and as a vital link to the community for women who had few social contacts at community level. They were embraced equally by all older mothers in this study, irrespective of career accomplishment. Young achievers, however, tended to rely on family and friends for support and did not attach the same level of importance to 'mothers' group'. For many of the study's older participants these groups provided a link to the community in which they lived. Many, especially career women, scarcely knew their neighbours, often despite living at the same address for many years. Laura explains:

There wasn't really anyone around here, certainly the lady across the road has 2 little kids but she's in and out all the time and everybody else is quite elderly and they do what they do!

For Harriet, mothers' group offered her an opportunity to meet other people socially:

And just socially the mothers' group and meeting other people, that's been good, because having moved to Melbourne when I was in my thirties, not having lived here in my twenties I didn't really know socially, as many people.

Although the new mothers' groups encompassed approximately 4-8 sessions led by M&CHNs, most groups continued to meet up socially, in one another's homes or other venues. For many, the groups allowed access to other new mothers living close by and were valuable to the women as a source of information. Mothers also described valuing the groups for the access they provided to children of similar ages. Cassie [career woman] explains:

We still meet! We're meeting today as we speak! And there's an immediate friendship for Jackson there! It's great, there's one [mother] over there [across the street] and another on this street behind...I'll show you a photo, [of the children of the group] it's very funny, somehow they know that they're kids ...

For Annie [dream-come-true] the mothers' group was a source of social outings and access to other mothers:

We'll go to a 'babes in arms' movie ...we do that in the mothers' group, we do that actually next week ... we can walk to some girls' houses and it's nice to go up to the shops and I'll bump into somebody I'd know and that's lovely, I didn't know anyone. I met one of the girls last week and we went and had a coffee.

For some, again principally career women, this access served as a useful source of reference and women describe learning from other mothers. Margaret [career woman], for example, found that younger mothers were more 'physical' with their infants and she tried to emulate their more relaxed demeanour:

I noticed we were all sitting there and we were much more conservative when we started and they [younger Mums] were quite physical with the baby throwing it around and that kind of reminded me that I should try to be more like that too and I try to throw Harry around more and to be more relaxed, I think that's a downside, you can be a bit stiffer if you're older. There's that thing where I don't want people to think I'm not looking together ...that I have to be well groomed ...

New mothers' groups also performed an important social role as a source of advice and reassurance, when a baby was unwell or suffering from some minor ailment. Annie [dream-come-true] describes her experience of her infant's gastro-enteritis:

And the next day threw up everywhere again and his nappies were really bad, so I rang the health centre and they said it might be the milk. To try soymilk, so I popped him in the pram and walked round to the shops and by the time we got back he'd soiled everything! It was dreadful! A couple of the girls in mothers' group said they had that as well! So I asked around 'what've you done? How long did it last?' She said a good week and you'd need paw paw for his bottom and everything.

Although there is a limited body of literature addressing the utility of first-time parent groups, as run by M&CHNs, searches revealed a study by Scott, Brady and Glynn (2001), examining first mother groups, in two centres in urban Melbourne. Scott et al. found that most mothers valued the interaction of the groups, both for themselves and for their children and, additionally, found that the majority of groups grew into "self sustaining social networks" (2001, p. 28). The role of the M&CHN in providing support to the individual mother receives more attention in the literature and several articles evaluating M&CHN support were accessed. Tarkka, Paunonen and Laippala (1999) found that first-time mothers' coping with childcare was affected by the social support received from their social network and from the public health nurses at child welfare clinic. Authors Borjesson, Paperin and Lindell (2004), who surveyed 120 mothers attending 60 child health clinics in Sweden, found that new mothers needed to be 'confirmed' into their mothering role. Although there is no indication of maternal ages, or indeed socio-economic status of the participants, in any of the above-mentioned studies, it raises the suggestion that both M&CHNs and new parent groups play important roles in supporting new mothers. As an extension of this theme, Logsdon and Davis (2003), who considered pregnancy and postpartum support among a broad range of Canadian and American mothers, found an association between adequate social support, less risky behaviour and less postnatal depression.

In sum, although the impact of social support for older mothers is not well addressed, the existing literature suggests clearly that, for mothers of all ages, adequate support mediates maternal adjustment and this holds especially true for women with few social resources (Navaie-Waliser, Martin, Tessaro, Campbell & Cross, 2000). Thus, it follows that for primiparae over 35, often with few social networks, new parent groups and M&CHNs may indeed form a vital link to the community. Scott et al. (2001) describe this link as "building a little village", thus nurturing community and social networks for the new mother (p. 29). In addition to identifying a lack of support as negatively impacting on mothering, many participants considered returning to work as a source of angst and this trend was seen especially for mothers returning to full-time work earlier than 6 months postpartum.

Maternal employment

Returning to work

By six months postpartum, eight career women in this study had returned to work (50%), although only 4 were working full-time, despite most planning pre-natally to do so. At this stage, none of the dream-come-true mothers were working and of four young achievers, three had returned to work 4-5 days per week. The fourth planned a year's maternity leave and the fifth was lost to follow-up. Overall, there was a tendency among career women in this study to have considerably revised earlier plans to work full-time and many had also extended their return to work deadlines. Of career women who had returned to full-time work, all had continued to breastfeed and express milk, despite the considerable effort involved. Young achievers, in general, did not display such revision of return to work plans and all three women returned to full-time work had ceased breastfeeding. None expressed milk.

Career women and work

For career women, a return to full-time work was not accompanied by any lessening of domestic or mothering duties and many described 'barely getting through each day' as they struggled to 'do it all'. All felt stressed and exhausted. Laura explains:

189

Some days it's just so exhausting, like I sit down and I go 'I don't know how I got through today'! And I don't know if I'm going to get up off this chair, just exhaustion to the point that you just feel that you're going to have a physical / mental breakdown ... I just cope with it, I don't know, just burst into tears or something which I think is equally ridiculous and other times ... like, if I'm at work I think 'I cannot deal with one more problem, I think I just have to get through until 6 o' clock or whatever, then I can go home and not think ... I worry about being able to do it all, every day I do! I wake up in the morning and go, God! What do I have to do today? You do all this and go to work and do all that and you come home and not be totally useless which I am honestly, a lot of the time, I'm not very good company ... I try not to feel that way ... I just drive in the driveway and I think 'oh my God, I don't even remember getting here!

Suzanne describes how she is 'barely hanging in', as she struggles to care for her twin boys and run her business from home. Her plans to have her twins cared for at a local childcare centre were thwarted by a lack of places, despite placing them on a waiting list well in advance of birth. Now, she employs someone to come in and care for the boys when she works and, although the arrangement is neither reliable nor regular, she continues to work as best she can.

I had one afternoon I was really flat chat, I had phone-calls and stuff and it was a drama I had to deal with and they just cried full on and I wasn't even able to get any one to come in, so I could stay away from them. I thought they need someone that's not stressed. I just wanted them to be looked after and I'm on the phone and people are saying 'oh the babies are crying!' and I'm thinking 'of course they are!' [throws her hands in the air] [Laughter] what! Do you think I'm deaf! [Laughter] good grief! ... Like, I have a really, really busy day tomorrow and I've been keeping it down, I'll start worrying about it tonight and I really have to keep it down, because if I started now I wouldn't get through today.

In addition to describing their lives as exhausting and stressful, career women often expressed feeling removed from their infants.

190

Feeling removed from the infant/s

Some mothers described feeling displaced in their mothering role and their centrality to the infant by having to relinquish care to a third party. There was a tendency towards feeling guilty too and recognition of social discourses dictating the importance of primary mothering. Gayle [career woman] explains:

I've felt a bit disconnected at times and I think you can get that way when you're taking her to childcare, removed. You know these days when I'm at home and I'm with her and I think, you look different from when I last looked at you properly, you see the thing is I don't look at her all day like I used to and I am that bit more removed too, because when Mark is here I want him to have that and what's happening now is that she's spending more time with him than with me. I'm realising that I've taken her away out of my life. I think part of it is this whole concept of the guilt and getting over that! If you put the child in childcare, you've got to give over the feeding, you know, everything to them [to the child carers] 3 or 4 days a week and then you read all these things that tell you you're terrible for doing it!

Laura also describes feeling she is not 'doing her job properly' in relinquishing the task of child raising principally to her mother:

I feel guilty every day when I go to work and I send Emily off to Mum, I really do ... she gets to see her cousins and she has much more fun than I do and her grandparents love having her and she loves being with them, but I feel it's my job I just think, you know. My Mum did her job and she's doing my job as well ... I suppose it comes from me and my expectations of what I should be doing, ... my mother from when she had us didn't work...

Changing priorities

Most career women described a change in priorities around work as mothering became increasingly important in their lives. Prior to birth, work had occupied a very central position in the lives of these women, but at this stage, shifting priorities gave rise to different emphases. Mothers now spoke of mothering as the 'most important thing' in their lives, similar to Leonard's (1993) description of mothering as a "world transforming" event (p. viii). This marks a significant departure from earlier

191

views of mothering as an add-on to the lives of the participants. Now women described feeling that it was 'just not worth it' to continue to work full-time. For some, this shift in priorities also included recognition that previous work commitments were untenable in light of changed responsibilities. Margaret [career woman] explains:

Mainly I realised that I couldn't do my old job again, at this stage, it would just be too demanding, managing people and situations, I can't walk in and walk out of it ... I was sort of on call, ... so I started to realise I couldn't do it, but also I don't want to do it. I don't know that I can do it very well and I don't know that I can be bothered with other people's problems ... I started thinking, I've got enough on my mind for now!

For Petra, this meant being quite clear about how much work she could offer her firm:

I've started to go back and do a little bit of work. I only do it for 4 or 5 hours, I think I can't cope too well with the pressure with the job that might fit in. It's such a deadline driven industry and because I feel obligated to try to get things finished ... and I suppose it's coming to terms with, they've got to realise and I've got to realise that no, we can't do that anymore and the amount of hours I can offer them is only so much...

Many, like Petra, found working or completing work at home to fit in around the infant's needs, to be a suitable compromise:

It's sort of worked out the past few days that I've done the work and I've brought the laptop home and once he's gone asleep I've worked like from 8- midnight and done the rest of the work, so I've done it that way...

Just not worth it

Although many of the career women had expended considerable energy and time working their way up to a position of seniority, some now questioned if it was indeed worth the sacrifice to continue to work long hours and have little time for family. There was a growing understanding that it might matter less in the 'grand scheme of things' than they had thought formerly. Laura explains:

192

I spent a lot of time and energy and ambition to get to my position, but really is it worth it, in the scheme of things, I just think someone else will do that job and at the end of the day no one will really care!

Laura further discusses moving house and simplifying her life, as a means of making more time for family and leisure. This marks a major departure from her earlier views of the importance of work:

I think I've actually changed because, because we're just debating selling here and getting something with a little less maintenance so we can have our weekends to ourselves and do things with Emily but his [husband's] view is that if we do that I would really have to give up working in the city, because he thought it would take more time away which is not the idea. And I think well, actually, you know, I'm quite open to that idea and he said if I asked you that 2 years ago you wouldn't do it ... you know, because it was important what you were doing and actually that's very true!

This trend of changing maternal priorities from work to child receives some attention in the literature addressing mothers and work and seems to relate particularly to older and more professional mothers. Smith-Pierce (1994), who studied middle-class mothers aged 35-40, found a shift in priorities from career to child and Leonard (1993) found that the meaning of work, for mothers in her study, was altered by the life-changing characteristics of new maternity. Brannen and Moss (1991), in their study of 255 working mothers, across a range of socio-economic classes and categories of employment, discovered that a substantial percentage of mothers who had planned to return to full-time work, later reduced hours or left the full-time position for a less stressful position elsewhere.

Part-time work / best of both worlds

At this stage, most mothers sought a balance between work and family life, similar to that described in chapter 6. Women who had managed to reduce hours of work, or continued to work from home in a part-time capacity, expressed greatest satisfaction with their circumstances. For Anthea [career woman], keeping her business 'ticking over' from home represented the best of both worlds:

Eric and I were talking about it the other night and we were sort of saying 'what is it worth doing? Is it worth keeping the business ticking over or' ... I said look! I feel I'm getting the

*best of everything at the moment so I don't get myself stressed and bombarded with work
and obviously, I'm only doing part time, that's what I want to do, keep the business going,
have a couple of kids.*

Little support at work

For career women returning to full-time work, particularly those returning to positions in deadline
driven industries, there was little available support in the work place. Some women describe prevailing
attitudes of 'if you want it all, then do it all' and further describe feeling uncomfortable displaying
infant photos at work, or even discussing the infant. There is a sense of having to attend to baby-related
duties furtively and mothers describe 'sneaking' away to phone child-carers or to express milk. Here,
Laura [career woman] describes how her work life is virtually unchanged, the only difference being
that she must try to express milk during her work breaks and must do so in a bathroom:

*When I go to work, the main thing that I take with me in terms of being a mother is having
to express, if that wasn't there my life at work hasn't changed, ... I express at work, in the
toilet, there's an area just off my office, shower bathroom and I try and use that, but every
now and then I run into one of the partners who goes for a jog about then, we don't
actually have a designated area, quite often I'm thinking this is ridiculous, I'm sitting on
the toilet, trying to express, looking at my watch thinking I've got a meeting in 20 minutes!*

Gayle [career woman] an academic, continued to breastfeed her infant, cared for on campus, though
she met with little support from either work or childcare:

*When I'm at work every couple of hours I have to think about feeding her or call them and
I come from my office and I feed her ... they were really against encouraging it in the
beginning, but you see I fed and I was the only one in both these places that does it, [work
or childcare] believe it or not, which I was amazed about!*

There was a tendency to feel that work often spilled over into the woman's domestic life, though the
reverse was seldom true. Jane [career woman] explains:

My life at work impinges more on my life at home than my life at home ever impinges on my work. I'll quite often be doing some work weekends or whatever and I feel that's not fair because on the other side very rarely ... bring anything from here or make excuses, 'can't do, or haven't done or whatever, because of what I do here.

Interestingly, Laura [career woman] describes lesser achieving women in her workplace as eliciting more tolerance from employers, than women in advanced roles:

I had to laugh the other day one of the secretaries came in at like 10.30 and it was because her cat kept her awake all night! Laughter, I had to leave the room as I was on the verge of saying something. I thought this will not sound very nice if you say it. I just went and sat down and thought 'now why did that not seem very fair to me? [Laughter] I wasn't going to make an issue of it, on the one hand I am a manager and she is not, but just the fact that she said 'my cat kept me awake last night so I had to have a couple of extra hours! That's why I'm late!

It's not fair / I have to do everything

Similar to that described in Chapter 6, older women in this study, continued to feel they carried the burden of overseeing the smooth running of the home and childcare. Anthea explains how she has to 'set her husband up' to look after the infant, although her husband is unemployed at the moment and she is working from home:

I've got to do work at the moment and I said to Eric, could you mind him Friday? You know how it is, I'm the one looking over him all the time, whereas if you could just do the feed and hand him [baby] over to someone else, but you don't [hand him over] and it just doesn't [work]...

Gayle [career woman] describes her experience of having to think about everything:

The hardest thing for me is that I have to think about everything for Tina and I have to run this house, Mark does none of it really ... even to think about paying the cleaner and

195

leaving the money out on the side, to actually going to the bank, Mark won't say to me have you got $60 for the cleaner today.

This trend of double maternal burden is commonly discussed in the literature surrounding maternity and work, particularly the feminist literature, and is reviewed in some detail at a later stage of this chapter.

Comparison with young achievers

In general, younger mothers in this study returning to full-time work tended to be pragmatic and displayed less angst than older mothers, around juggling both work and family. These younger women had mostly grown up in homes where their own mothers had worked and they tended to look back to their upbringing and feel that they had not suffered as a result of maternal absence. When I enquired of these women about their return to work experiences, the responses fell into three main categories: just doing what I have to do, no real dilemma about working and mothering as a part of life / not making it a chore.

Just doing what I have to do

Among the women whose pregnancies had been unplanned, there was a sense of managing as best they could with the circumstance in which they found themselves. Financial imperatives often dictated return to work dates, rather than personal choice.

For Madeleine, the baby's earlier than expected arrival and her husband's work circumstances conspired to send her back to work earlier than anticipated:

Money was the only issue, we had setbacks that we hadn't expected, we hadn't been planning to have the baby you know and then when she was born she was in hospital for 3 weeks and we hadn't expected that and Scott took three weeks off and where Scott was working wasn't doing very well, so I had to go back to work.

No real dilemma about working

In general, young achievers described no real dilemma in working and did not seem troubled by the same degree of angst or guilt as older mothers. Most saw no contradiction in juggling working and family life and some, in fact, felt their lives were considerably easier than their contemporaries of two decades ago. Anita explains how much tougher her mother's circumstances were:

I think it was much harder for women 20/30 years ago, take my mother, she had 4 kids and she was working too, you don't have that nowadays. My mother says she would just come home give the baby a bottle on the couch and he could drink it, she had 4 [children] and working full-time and all the cooking and cleaning... I'm not really worried about being back to work, she'll cry but you know they have to get used to it...

For some young achievers, used to having their own money and contributing to the household finances, feeling dependent on spousal income, even temporarily, was an unpleasant experience. Melanie, describes returning to work as something of a relief:

I'm actually quite relieved to be going back to work and also because I'm not depriving him and I will work on weekends. That will give Alan one on one time with him, and that's really important ... the big thing was because I'd always contributed to the finances [household] suddenly not contributing was really hard, so even though I was looking after him and keeping house that was really hard, so going back, I felt better about it ...

Mothering as part of life / not making it a chore
Among the young achievers, proximity to other children and being close to one's natal family seemed together to predict greater maternal adaptation and less likelihood of 'making mothering a chore'. This attitude is in contrast with the tendency towards mothering as a conscious activity, described by career mothers in chapter 5. Here
Madeleine [young-achiever] explains her pragmatic approach:

I've had a lot to do with small kids and I made a conscious effort not to let it be a chore to let it get to me, not to be fussy too, I didn't want to be ... like I've had girlfriends, like you'll make a date to go for a coffee and they'll cancel, the baby's asleep, sorry! And apart from the fact that you are making your own life difficult, you're putting other people out as well and you lose friends ... I think people make it difficult for themselves by expecting that they have to vacuum 4 times a day, ... I've never been one for routine routine, she sleeps when she's tired, I don't quite understand this [obsession with routine] ... if I think she's really tired I'll put her in the cot and she will go to sleep ...

Kim, too, endorsed a common-sense approach and viewed the baby as part of family life:

I guess I've been lucky and I know that not all babies are the same, but I still wonder. I think a lot of it is still to do with the parents, just common sense and this thing, 'but I need quiet time with my husband', I don't see why special time with your husband needs to be exclusive, you can still have a cup of coffee and talk, they're [babies] not intrusive at this stage. If she's grumpy we'll put her to bed, if she's happily playing we'll leave her ...

In general, younger mothers of this study, were less likely to feel troubled by the burden of having to 'do everything', as older mothers described. One possible explanation may relate to a greater tolerance among younger mothers when tasks were performed to less than exacting standards. This group of women may also have been more direct in insisting on assistance from their partners. Madeleine explains her approach:

I just get Scott and say right, it's your turn!

Discourse and the literature around mothers and work

Despite current female employment trends and an increasing need for dual income to maintain living standards, mother discourses embrace two competing strands, advocating that mothers should ideally stay-at-home to care for their children, particularly during infancy (Hays, 1996) and also that women should work (Filene, 1998). Although it could be argued that individual mothers could simultaneously embrace both strands with differing intensities, the existence of competing discourses, in my opinion, intensifies the angst contemporary mothers experience as they attempt to do it all. Notions of intensive, all-consuming mothering (Hays, 1996), discussed in chapter 2, prevail. On the other hand, mothering only continues to be a socially devalued role and professional status is more highly regarded (Hoffnung, 1995). The revolution in women's workforce participation, in terms of what sort and amount of paid work women might engage in, has led to a veritable explosion of literature, exploring the effects of maternal employment on the well being of mothers and children. This trend has been particularly evident since the 1980s.

Literature addressing maternal employment is extensive and varied, but in general falls into two broad categories: studies comparing outcomes in the children of employed versus non-employed mothers (Gottfried & Gottfried, 1988; Gross et al., 2001; Hoffman & Youngblade, 1999; Stein & Susser, 2000; Zybert et al., 1978) and, to a lesser extent, studies assessing the maternal well-being of employed mothers (Brannen & Moss, 1991; Eyer, 1996; Gjerdingen, McGovern, Bekker & Willemsen, 2000; Granrose & Kaplan, 1996; Hattery, 2001; Hochschild, 1989). Interestingly, studies examining the effects of maternal employment on children do not support the negative view endorsed by social discourses, for example: Gottfried and Gottfried (1988); Gross et al. (2001); Hoffman and Youngblade (1999); Stein and Susser (2000) and Zybert et al. (1978), all supported equal or better outcomes among children of employed mothers. In the current study, work-associated issues, as articulated by the mothers, related principally to maternal stress and guilt, finding a balance between work and family, and, to a lesser extent, breastfeeding among employed mothers. A comparison of the literature relating to these themes is presented here.

Maternal work, stress and guilt

Hattery (2001) examined the work-related experiences of 30 mothers with young children, age and socio-economic circumstance unspecified, and found that women fell into four broad categories: conformists, who tended to stay-at-home with children, despite the financial sacrifice involved; non-conformists, who were motivated to continue to work by feeling a need to provide economically for their children and who also felt they had a right to work for personal satisfaction; pragmatists, who sought high standards of fulfilling work but suffered tremendous guilt around juggling family; and innovators, who sought to create ways to preserve work, finances and family balance. The career women of this study who elected to return to full-time work did so for a variety of reasons, including personal fulfilment and career imperatives, and most probably would have been considered by Hattery (2001), above, to be pragmatists. Undeniably, they suffered tremendous guilt around childcare. The younger women, also returning to full-time work, did not seem to suffer from the same degree of angst and most probably fitted into Hattery's non-conformist group, citing financial imperatives as the prime motivating force in their return to work plans, but also expecting to work for personal fulfilment.

Leonard (1993), who studied stress and coping in the transition to parenthood of first-time mothers with career commitments (n = 18), similarly found that stresses associated with returning to work were alleviated by financial necessity and meaningful employment.

In general, a return to work prior to six months postpartum is considered especially stressful (Leonard, 1993), particularly for mothers who work in unsupportive work settings. McGovern et al. (1997), widely published in the field of employed mothers' postpartum health, found that maternity leave over 6 months was associated with improved maternal outcomes. Indeed, maternal stress and guilt are frequently paired with maternal employment (Erlandsson & Eklund, 2003; Gjerdingen et al., 2000; Leucken, Suarez, Kuhn, Barefoot, Blumental, Siegler & Williams, 1997; Rankin, 1993), particularly full-time work (Brannen & Moss, 1991; Olson & DiBrigida, 1994). Leukin et al. (1997) compared the effects of parental status (defined as having children at home) on working mothers (n = 109). They found increased rates of home strain among working mothers, evidenced by higher levels of excreted cortisol. Hochschild (1989) also found that many working mothers initially tried to function as 'super moms' simultaneously doing most household chores, caring for the infant and participating in paid employment. Many felt crushed by their workload. Eyer (1996), whose writings address cultural expectations and maternal guilt, discusses additional stresses for working mothers. She postulates that 'mommy wars' raging in parenting and women's magazines put women in impossible positions of wanting to do 'everything' and to do it all well. Eyer further suggests that discourses of the working mother pits stay-at-home mothers against mothers who work, by peddling "double messages" about careers and choice for working women (p. 107).

Successive authors have also found that mothering, per se, is not the principal source of angst for working mothers, but rather the ancillary domestic concerns that go with being a mother. Rankin (1993), who conducted a study of 118 employed mothers, found that maternal stresses included principally a lack of time and maternal guilt around the child. Child-related problems also contributed. Others found that maternal stress related to social circumstances, for example, Erlandsson and Eklund (2003) found that stresses endured by working mothers related to their 'social and temporal contexts', rather than work alone. Lambden (2001) felt that a woman's perceived self-efficacy affected her subsequent integration of her multiple roles as worker and mother. More startling was Gelles and Hargreaves (1981) finding, of higher levels of maternal violence associated with working mothers' excessive domestic responsibilities. This broad-ranging American study (n = 1146) found correlates between low socio-economic status and violent maternal behaviour.

In contrast, Canadian Roxburgh (1997) found that working mothers (n = 500) were significantly less stressed that their non-mothering colleagues, in the presence of job control and partner support. Abrams and Jones (1997) examined the impact of multiple roles in a working mother's life among women from the University of Chigago's Women's Business Group (n = 104). They found an inverse relationship between the number of roles that a career mother assumed and the level of psychological distress the mother felt. They postulate that this trend relates to the broader social contact such women enjoyed (p. 19). Secret's (1994) survey found no correlation between maternal work status and maternal well being (n = 983).

Finding a balance between work and family

For the women of this current study, particularly career women, part-time work was seen as the best of everything and resulted in a lesser expression of maternal guilt. Of the eight career women who had or intended to return to full-time work, all but two would have preferred to work fewer hours and were unhappy when unable to do so. This finding of maternal satisfaction in balancing work and family as being related to preferred working hours is supported by Brannen and Moss (1991). In their English study of 255 working mothers, Brannen and Moss found that a congruence between preferred maternal work and preferred number of working hours augured well for maternal satisfaction (pp. 130-135). Mahony (1995), meanwhile, discussed the difficulties for women of juggling work and family, and made mention of a preponderance of part-time workers among self-employed women, particularly mothers of pre-school children. For Mahony, this trend contributed to women's lesser earning potential. In this study, financial concerns were of lesser importance than making time for family and several women creatively addressed their difficulties by setting up consultancies to work part-time from home.

This balance between work and family is a complex one, and seems to be informed by a variety of influences. In this study, career women's views of appropriate parenting seemed to be largely informed by prevalent mother discourses. In general, these women subscribed to the model of intensive mothering described by Hays (1996) and criticised by Thurer (1994), as causing maternal angst by reminding the mother of the "portentousness of her responsibility" (p. 260). Many mothers made decisions about balancing work and family, based on culturally acceptable practices and also on personal beliefs about appropriate parenting, and this finding is commonly expressed in the literature (Hattery, 2001; Hays, 1996; Walzer, 1998). Peters (1998) also discusses anxiety in working mothers as related to a fear of being unable to simultaneously "inhabit two worlds" (p. 73), which is similar to the angst expressed by older mothers in this study and in direct contrast to the more pragmatic views expressed by the younger mothers.

201

Double burden

In the current study, many career women described feeling over-burdened by having responsibility for the smooth running of the home and overseeing childcare arrangements, while continuing to work as before the infant was born. Most accommodated the additional burden by working late into the night, in order that the infant would not be deprived of maternal time. Many had husbands who worked long hours and thus did not contribute particularly to domestic / childrearing activities. A similar trend is found within the literature. In general, limited spousal participation in childcare and domestic activities and limited spousal support are well recognised as contributing to the role strain many working mothers suffer (Brannen & Moss, 1991; Hattery, 2001; Hewlett, 2002b; Hochschild, 1989; Lerner, 1994; Pleck, 1985). There is also a suggestion that women bear primary responsibility for child care and household tasks even when actively engaged in careers (Apter, 1993; Deutsch, 1999; Glenn, 1994; Granrose & Kaplan, 1996; Hattery, 2001; Hewlett, 2002b; Weingarten, 1994). In this study, of mothers engaged in full-time work, a disproportionate sharing of domestic work was often troublesome and is comparable to that discussed by Gornick and Meyers (2003). Hochschild (1989) also found that working mothers in her study attended to most of the domestic and childcare work at home and were unhappy about having to do so. Nonetheless, they were reluctant to create marital friction by insisting on getting help from their spouse. For older mothers in this study, particularly for women who considered they had egalitarian relationships with their partners, gender role allocation of chores came as something of a surprise. Most recent studies confirm these findings, for instance, Hewlett (2002b), in her sterling work on the dilemmas of career and family, concurred with this view and describes traditional division of labour at home as troublesome for many contemporary high-achieving women.

By comparison, younger mothers, in the current study, did not describe the same level of angst around working full-time and, although the very small sample precludes any generalisations, several tendencies are noted. Each of the younger mothers who returned to full-time work had taken steps to minimise her other burdens, had ceased breastfeeding and had enlisted the assistance of family / partner in managing domestic / childcare chores. Most made conscious efforts 'not to make a chore' out of mothering, as distinct from older mothers who tended to want to 'do it properly'. This differing maternal attitude between older and younger mothers in this study may relate to the fact that most of the younger women had grown up in homes where their own mothers had been employed. These women anticipated no conflict between work and mothering roles. In contrast, older mothers had mostly been the recipients of full-time mothering and may thus have different expectations. Another possible explanation may perhaps relate to the extensive reading engaged in by older professional mothers, which may contribute to an increased awareness of negative social discourses around working mothers. This may in turn influence levels of angst and guilt.

Breastfeeding and maternal employment

In general, the literature supports an association between lower duration of breastfeeding and a return to work, particularly full-time work (Auerbach, 1990; Baiagioli, 2003; Corbett-Dick & Bezek, 1997; Earland, Ibrahim & Harpin, 1997; Frank, 1998; Hill, Humenick, Argubright & Aldag, 1997; Kearney & Cronenwett, 1991). The timing of return to work is also implicated, with the women returning earliest, faring least well (Rojjanasrirat, 2000). Although the overall picture of breastfeeding continuance patterns among working mothers looks bleak, there is a clear suggestion of greater breastfeeding continuance rates among middle-class professional women. Americans Visness and Kennedy (1997) conducted a wide-scale survey among postpartum women (n = 9953) and found that highest rates of breastfeeding continuance occurred among 'white professional women'. Kurinij, Shiono, Ezrine, and Rhoads (1989), also in the U.S.A., conducted a large-scale survey of maternal employment and breastfeeding duration, contrasting the experiences of black (n = 668) and white (n = 511) women, across a range of social circumstances. They too found that white women in professional occupations had the longest duration of breastfeeding. Bagwell, Kendrick, Stitt, Leeper, Espy and Gedel, (1992) found that breastfeeding duration was "related positively and independently to increased maternal age and parity" (p. 205). Meanwhile, Berryman (1991) and Berryman et al. (1999) also found higher rates of breastfeeding among older mothers compared to younger mothers. Hill (2000) learnt that the highest rates of breastfeeding related to increased maternal age over 35, college-education and annual income over US $25,000. Finally, a host of studies have linked higher rates of breastfeeding to higher maternal education (Chezem, Friesen & Boettcher, 2003; Hill, 2000; Lawson & Tulloch, 1995).

In this study, breastfeeding trends were not entirely typical, though a high percentage of career women continued to breastfeed at six months postpartum, including all four women who had returned to full-time work before this time. This rate of eleven out of sixteen (69%) is higher than the national average of 44-50% at 6 months (ABS, 2003b; National Center for Epidemiology and Population Health, [NCEPH] 1998). Of career women who had ceased breastfeeding, all cited insufficient supply as the reason for weaning the infant, as discussed in chapter 5. Three out of four young achievers had ceased breastfeeding, citing 'too much hassle' as the principal reason, and this finding is at odds with prevalent associations of maternal education and socio-economic status as positively influencing continuance rates. Of the dream-come-true mothers, only one mother continued to feed at six months and the most commonly cited reason for cessation was 'insufficient milk'.

Prohibitive and unsympathetic work practices were found to influence breastfeeding duration for the younger mothers, and such practices are recognised within the literature as exerting an inhibiting influence on breastfeeding continuance rates (Baiagioli, 2003; Frank, 1998; Visness & Kennedy, 1997). The opposite of this trend is to be seen in Norway, where breastfeeding continuance trends of approx 80% at 6 months postpartum are seen, irrespective of maternal employment status, postulated to be a direct result of sympathetic work practices (Alvarez, 2003).

Until this point, the discussion has centred principally on maternal experience as understood by the mothers in this study. Now, the social implications of later timing of pregnancy are briefly revisited, and the mothers' understandings and experiences of social expectations around maternity are discussed. This discussion aims to locate social conceptions of older mothering and to form a basis for comparison of focus group findings [Appendix C].

Social implications of later timing of pregnancy

Social timing of pregnancy is commonly held to be related to social mores, and there is generally strong social approval for giving birth within appropriate time-lines (Daniels & Weingarten, 1982; Hoffnung, 1995). Daniels and Weingarten (1982) further suggest a common social understanding of the right time to become a parent, which in Australia is around thirty years of age, similar to statistical averages (ABS, 2003a). Considerable evidence suggests that women choosing to delay childbearing beyond social norms may feel 'out of time' with their peers (Dobrzykowski & Stern, 2003; Neurgarten & Datan, 1973; Rossi, 1980). Additionally, women electing to delay childbearing beyond 35 years are often portrayed as selfish and aberrant in their behaviour (Hoffnung, 1995; Kaplan, 1992).

In this study, women described understanding their timing of pregnancy as considerably later than societal norms of approximately 30 years for a first baby. For most, this awareness of time 'running out' invested the experience with a level of urgency and led to anxiety about 'getting it right'. Others felt victim to 'public scrutiny' and felt there was no margin for error as an older mother. Jennifer [dream-come-true] explains:

> *It's amazing how many people say 'she's young' [indulgently], but when you're an older Mum, its really like you should know better!*

204

In the next section, maternal social expectations and beliefs are discussed. These expectations presented in three categories, as follows: following the social order; social approval for childbearing, and finally, mixed messages about mothering.

Following the social order

Many women in this study arrived at the marriage stakes considerably later than peers. Career women particularly, even within stable partnered or marital relationships, frequently postponed childbearing for quite some time. Several spoke of their families 'giving up on them' ever-becoming parents. When they eventually became pregnant, it was a cause for family celebration and several women speak of their families wholeheartedly embracing this late but 'normal' following of the social order, of marriage and children. Cassie [career woman] explains:

Well, when you've been single for such a long time, getting married and having children is normal and your parents think there's something wrong when you're not and when all of a sudden when you're married and having children you're more set to their pattern.

Embracing the social order of marriage and family was greeted with social approval, and the women of this study basked in their new state of belonging. Similar to the participants in Dobrzykowski and Stern's (2003) study, participants, particularly career women, believed that although they had followed the "sentimental order of society a little late" their greater life experience balanced their late arrival at mothering (p. 249). Although the majority of women in this study had electively postponed parturition, some, principally mothers of the dream-come-true group, felt that their situation had been misinterpreted socially. These women were distressed to be associated with women who had 'selfishly chosen' to delay childbearing. Jennifer [dream-come-true] explains:

People never understand, they think it's all about choice ... they automatically think that you have chosen to leave it this long to have a baby, ... See in our case, which is probably unusual, I didn't meet Ian till I was older, we didn't get married till we were 37 so we've only been married 2 years, it's just things like, people do tend to have this attitude well, you are selfish because you have chosen to do this ... there's such negativity towards an older mum.

Soial approval

In general, social approval of pregnancy and mothering came as something of a surprise, and participants of this study described a transformation from previous anonymity to the centre of social attention. Many spoke of now feeling part of their community, which in turn was described as taking on the feel of a rural village. Others discussed their surprise at realising that they, as mothers, were viewed differently by friends and acquaintances. Harriet explains her surprise:

It's been interesting from a social point of view ... a lot of people say that when you become a parent, you meet a lot of other people at school things and kinder and that, it's another dimension. I think it's interesting that some of my sister's friends who I've been friends with and who have children, they see me differently, that's been a bit of a surprise.

For the majority of the older mothers, irrespective of career accomplishment, this social approval of mothering was unexpected and women talk of attracting attention when at the shops or out walking with the baby. Kerri [career woman] explains:

When you walk down the street with a baby everybody talks to you!

Some like Jane [career woman] basked in a glow of maternal pride when a stranger admired her infant:

People are a lot more ... I get a lot more smiles from people, with Keegan and in fact some people, I've gotten stopped by someone, I thought I was in her way, this woman came up to me and Keegan and said 'excuse me' and I said 'I'm sorry' oh no, she said, 'I just wanted to tell you your baby is just a beautiful boy, it is a boy, isn't it'? I said 'yeah' and she said 'he's just gorgeous and they didn't have clothes like that when I had my children' and it was just amazing, I just sort of felt ... big chest pumped out ... before when you went shopping before you were pretty much anonymous unless it was someone you knew, but most people walked past you ... It actually is a bit more like going out in a country town, we get it more now, a lot more smiles and a lot more little comments ... yeah, a lot more compliments about me not looking my age now, its really good ... then it comes round to age and 'you're not, are you'? [not 43]

206

Although most women were aware of strong social approval for mothering and received attention and confirmation in their social roles as mothers, some, again particularly career women were also distressed at social devaluing of the mothering role.

Mixed messages about mothering

Social devaluing of stay-at-home mothering and conflicting expectations of paid work / mothering were experienced by several of the study participants, again particularly career women. Here, Abigail [career woman] admits to feeling annoyed when she found herself required to justify her maternal role and her lack of 'real work'. She explains:

> *I've been quite annoyed at times ... when people have said to me 'so what are you doing?.*
> *I ran into someone, an actor, I'd done a review of her plays and she [said] 'so, what writing*
> *have you been doing? What are you up too? I've got a pram, for God's sake! What are you*
> *up to? [angry] and I say [indicating the pram, with a flourish] this is what I've been doing!*

Some career women were aware of thwarting the social expectations of providing exclusive care for the infant in the early months by an early return to full-time work. These women described feeling criticised by others, particularly other women, for the choices they had made. This finding is similar to Eyer's suggestion that differing discourses set women in opposition to one another, by presenting "double messages about working mothers" (1996, p. 107). Laura [career woman] explains:

> *My sister and sisters in law, they'd say to me 'well, have you taken 12 months maternity*
> *leave? And I would say 'actually I haven't, I'm going back in April and you could almost*
> *hear the [gasp] not quite sense of approval ... I just, I suppose I sometimes get annoyed*
> *because I don't feel that everyone deserves an explanation, you know I've never questioned*
> *why you don't work, why you stay home all the time and why you do what you do ... I think*
> *that the assumption was that now you are having a baby so this is the expectation ... I think*
> *some women actually chose to do that [stay-at-home], but don't make allowances for*
> *people who don't chose to do that. Somehow because they have decided that they will stay*
> *home that they are actually making a much bigger sacrifice than you are, well I think it's*
> *just a choice and quite frankly I'm sure there are some women who have no desire to go*

out and work and that's OK too, but I think women still judge women much harsher than anyone else would!

Women of this study, again principally career women, often spoke of government suggestions to pay mothers to extend maternity leave as contributing to the angst suffered by working mothers. This move was seen as counter-productive and as likely to endorse extended maternity leave as the appropriate social action. Sally explains:

I think the government are sort of perpetuating that [the problem] by trying to pay women to stay-at-home instead of going back to the workforce, which seems to me quite strange, put it into day-care or something, it's something you can't find and it costs a fortune. It's almost like saying like you know, that we don't think its acceptable that you're taking jobs away from men or other people and you think 'how narrow minded is that' why should employers think any different, I just don't think it's an incentive to getting the workplace more friendly to people coming back to work after maternity leave.

Data from the focus groups present striking parallels to the mothers' understandings of prevalent maternal discourses and are discussed in Appendix C. Findings of requiring additional assistance with breastfeeding and 'ordinary' care of the infant display close resonance to concerns and suggestions articulated by the mothers of this study, in response to the question "in retrospect, what, if anything, would've helped with your experiences of mothering?" These suggestions are further explored in chapter 8.

Summary

In this chapter, the discussion has centred on four central issues. Firstly, issues surrounding maternal age and mothering identity were addressed. In this study, participants were found to have constructed an image of themselves as 'older mothers' rather than as mothers. This notion of age as occupying a central position in mothering experiences was found particularly among the accounts of career women. Secondly, the theme 'feeling like a mother, achieving the transition' has been explored, and although this theme of maternal satisfaction and pleasure in the mothering role is addressed within the literature, findings here are in contrast to other studies. In this study, four to six months postpartum was a more usual juncture for achieving maternal ease and comfort within the mothering role and this tendency was again most marked among career women. In contrast, maternal role achievement is commonly described in the literature at 3-4 months postpartum. However, despite a longer than usual time to adjustment, participants in this study were overwhelmingly positive about their mothering experiences by six to eight months postpartum and most described recommending it highly. At this stage, most had become confident mothers.

The third section of this chapter has discussed maternal employment, principally returning to work and balancing work and family. Similar to findings in the scant body of literature addressing this notion, this study found that having a baby was a 'world transforming' event for older mothers and prior expectations of mothering as a supplementary role were challenged, causing a re-negotiation of maternal self and life-goals.

Fourthly, a review of social discourses and expectations of appropriate mothering, as experienced by the mothers of this study, was also undertaken. Mothers here described feeling amazed to be the centre of social attention, which was in stark contrast to their previously anonymous position within the community. Conflict between competing social discourses for contemporary older mothers was also briefly discussed.

In chapter 8, conclusions from the study are presented and the significance of the current study is explored within the opportunity it presents to provide more meaningful maternal support for primiparae over 35. Unsustainable nursing practices, as they relate to casual and individual approaches to dilemmas presented by this group of mothers, are also presented, together with recommendations for practice.

CHAPTER 8

DISCUSSION AND RECOMMENDATIONS

This final chapter presents conclusions from the study "Transition to motherhood for first-time mothers aged 35 years and above" and sheds some light on the experiences of first-mothering, particularly the social context of mothering for this group of women. For primiparae over 35, early mothering is commonly regarded as a specially stressful time, above and beyond that experienced by most new mothers. Anecdotal evidence from midwives, maternal and child health nurses, doctors and other health professionals suggest that transition to motherhood for this group is fraught with difficulty, including a postulated increased incidence of postnatal depression and maternal maladjustment.

Additionally, as the age of childbearing women in Australia continues to rise and health care reforms dictate ever reducing hospital and community services, the implications for the health and well being of primiparae over 35 assume increasing importance. It is therefore imperative that health professionals learn as much as possible about the needs and concerns of these women in order to provide them with more meaningful maternal support. That knowledge and understanding has been the primary quest of this research study.

As expected, considerable anxiety was reported in the early days of mothering by the participants of this study and this trend was most marked among professional women. However, despite a shaky start, by six months postpartum most had become confident in their mothering abilities. Although these women used services and phoned for advice more than other mothers, they did not demonstrate the high levels of post-natal maladjustment or depression commonly associated with primiparae over 35. Participants of this study also identified a need for additional professional and social support during the early postpartum period. Nonetheless, findings here indicate that primiparous mothers over 35 years do well, despite expectations to the contrary. This study also found that transition to motherhood occurred over a longer time for participants than that discussed elsewhere.

The significance of the current study rests in the opportunity it presents to gain a greater insight into the experiences of maternity for older primiparae. It also presents a contribution to the intellectual debate surrounding the social context of modern older primiparity, a relatively new social phenomenon. Overall, it is clear that first-time mothers over 35 have concerns and needs that differ from other mothers. Close attention to the experiences of this study's participants may inform future nursing strategies and may thus mitigate transition issues experienced by this group of healthy women.

Recommendations for nursing and midwifery, as informed by the current study, are presented here to address those concerns.

This chapter presents six areas for discussion: an overview of the findings; the social context of contemporary older first mothering; contribution to the intellectual debate; feedback from participants; implications for nursing / midwifery practice; and finally, limitations of the study and recommendations for further study.

Importance of this study / contribution to existing literature

This study is important because of the insight it offers into the experience of first-time mothering over 35 years, a trend of global significance and a previously little researched subject. Australia, like its international counterparts, is exhibiting a trend towards later childbearing, and declining birth rates add to the social importance of individual children. This demographic shift towards older maternity has been evident for more than twenty years and continues to gain momentum in advanced industrial nations, particularly westernised nations. In 2002, in Australia, women aged 30-34 years recorded the highest number of births of any age group, for the third consecutive year. This trend represents a marked departure from earlier trends of younger maternal age (ABS, 2003a). At the same time, the birth-rate for women aged greater than 35 has more than doubled in the past two decades and a sizeable portion of this group are first-time mothers (ABS, 2003a). In addition to trends of later childbearing, current health care reforms result in reducing services. New trends of earlier discharge from hospital following birth, fewer community health services, and social trends of fewer precious children born later in life together contribute to the potential for social isolation of new mothers and contribute to the urgency surrounding maternity for these mothers. In this climate, the health and well being of primiparae over 35 and their infants is of great importance. Thus it is essential that health professionals learn as much as possible about the needs and concerns of this growing group of women, in order to better assist them in their transition to motherhood. Towards that end, the aim of this study was to explicate the experiences of older first-time mothers from pregnancy to approximately six to eight months postpartum and, in so doing, shed some light on the unique nature of these women and their maternal experiences. As such, this study adds to the scant body of literature addressing the experiences of older first-time mothers, particularly the social context of mothering for this group of healthy women.

One indication of how overdue this study was and how very limited is the literature on older primiparous mothering was brought home to me recently when I published a paper: 'The graying of the obstetric population, what implications for care' (Carolan 2003b). This article resulted in more than 200 requests for reprints from a wide variety of health care personnel, including: student midwives; medical students; doctors; midwives and maternal and child health nurses. Even more surprising were the several requests I have received via the Midwifery Research mailing list for information and advice for student midwifery curricula. I have also received a request from an American author, researching and writing a book on women's biological clocks. Thus it would seem, this qualitative study may add significantly to the sparse literature pool addressing the experiences of maternity for this growing group of women.

Overview of the findings / what is new to this study?

Many parallels are to be found among the experiences of this study's participants and those of all new mothers, particularly in regard to new maternity as a time of disruption, anxiety and chaos. However, there are also striking differences noted and new information uncovered in this study related to: anxiety and vigilance; doing it properly / mothering as a 'chore'; later than usual achievement of transition to motherhood; re-definition of 'self' as an older mother and finally, work and balance / confusing social messages. As we shall see, these findings are closely related to the five interweaving themes of this study, explicated in chapter 3. Those themes are:

- Vulnerability and anxiety
- The project 'doing it properly' / getting it right
- Finding my own way / challenging expectations
- The meaning of being an older mother
- The importance of work / balancing work and family

As the term 'interweaving' suggests, these themes, although separate, are to be found as an interlinking and underlying matrix among the findings of this study. As such it is not possible to deal with each theme in isolation and, as we shall see in the following overview, shades of the themes underpin each section for discussion.

Vulnerability and anxiety

In this study, anxiety was commonly displayed by older mothers, particularly professional women (Carolan, 2003c, in press-c). This anxiety was generally focused on the infant's perceived vulnerability, with several mothers considering their babies to be at increased risk of damage or dying during pregnancy, birth and the newborn period. This notion of infant vulnerability was generally not medically substantiated but persisted despite all the infants in this study being healthy term infants. It may relate, in part, to a common understanding among the study participants of pregnancy as an exceptional achievement (a miracle). Notions of infant vulnerability were most marked among women who had availed of IVF / fertility treatments, but were also noted among women who described their pregnancies as 'last chance'. Other contributing factors may relate to high levels of pregnancy surveillance and the allocation of 'at risk' category, as a consequence of advanced maternal age.

Despite considerable evidence to the contrary, the notion of age-associated increased medical risk prevails and, in this study, appears to have influenced pregnancy care for the participants. Many participants considered their pre-pregnancy health to be above average. However, on presenting for pregnancy care, they discovered that they were deemed to be at risk for a plethora of medical conditions. Increased pregnancy surveillance was common and often precipitated a domino effect of subsequent testing and re-testing. The women, well-educated, articulate and Internet literate, for their part often insisted on additional ultrasonic scans and genetic testing as reassurance for their perceived vulnerable pregnancy. Most were advised to attend a tertiary hospital for care. This may in part relate to medical concerns about litigation. For many participants, perceptions of 'high risk' pregnancy fuelled pre-natal concerns and seem to have resulted in an emotional distancing from the pregnancy. This in turn, coupled with late commencement of maternity leave, appears to have resulted in limited time for reflection, and many participants described feeling lost and ill-prepared when the infant arrived. A sense of feeling unprepared co-existed paradoxically with extensive preparation. Indeed, the women presented to midwifery and nursing staff as a curious paradox, as simultaneously assertive and vulnerable, and they were often considered a challenging group of mothers to care for. Pre-natal anxieties experienced by the mothers seemed to spill over into the neonatal period, resulting in a tendency towards vigilance in the new mother, which manifested in disproportionate concerns about infant illness and/or demise. Many mothers described being initially unable to sleep or to 'relax their guard' for weeks on end. Limited prior exposure to other children, social isolation as new mothers and fewer social and family supports may also have contributed to this situation, which seems considerably more intense in this study than that described elsewhere. Throughout this study, maternal approach to infant care was characterised by information gathering and planning, and this approach is discussed as follows.

The project 'doing it properly' / finding my own way

During pregnancy and prior to conception, mothers in this study undertook extensive literature searches and made elaborate plans for the infant's socialisation. Some, particularly career women, went to considerable effort to be fully informed in a bid to circumvent later difficulties and to understand 'what they were facing'. Limited prior exposure to children and a limited social network seemed to intensify the women's need for information. This trend of extensive reading continued during the early days of mothering and new mothers attempted to do 'everything properly' informed by their reading and preparation. For many, mothering was viewed as an overwhelming responsibility in which the mother had a limited opportunity to 'get it right'. The resulting maternal approach in this study was largely conscious and striving and mothering became something of a 'chore'. However, by four to six months, most participants had relaxed their approach and spoke of a dawning realisation of having to 'find my own way' and of realising that the infant was 'just a baby', rather than the enormous responsibility the infant had been until this point. At this stage, there was less emphasis on 'getting it right', though mothering continued to be a source of angst for many. Midwives and maternal and child health nurses spoke of such mothers making their own lives difficult by adhering to exacting standards. In contrast, both younger mothers and less accomplished older mothers in this study were more likely to embrace family life, and seemed to absorb infant care routines into their lives without 'making a fuss'. This theme of 'mothering as a chore' is seldom found in the literature relating to contemporary older mothering, though some mention of mothering as 'conscious and striving', is found. In addition to, and as a consequence of, mothering as an awesome responsibility, many mothers in this study described a later than usual transition, which has been addressed in chapters 6 and 7 and is briefly reviewed below.

Later than usual achievement of transition to motherhood

The literature surrounding transition to motherhood supports a general consensus of 3-4 months to achieving maternal identity and transition to motherhood. However, the findings of this study suggest a considerably longer time, which is interpreted here as related to a distancing from pregnancy, anxiety and perceptions of fetal / infant vulnerability. In this study, 4-6 months was a more usual time for participants to report 'finding my own way' and this trend of later maternal role attainment is not found in the literature. In tandem with later transition to motherhood, participants in this study articulated a clear phase of reflection on the meaning of maternal age, resulting in a redefinition of self, which is discussed as follows.

214

Re-definition of 'self' as an 'older mother'

Re-definition of self as an older mother is perhaps the most significant of the study's five major themes and advanced maternal age appears to have been especially significant to maternal identity among the mothers of this study. Participants frequently discussed the meaning of 'older maternal age' and the implications of maternal age both for themselves as mothers and for their infants, as the children of older mothers. Many prefaced sentences with 'as an older mother'. This thread presented in terms of risk perceptions during pregnancy and birth, as impressions of heightened vulnerability in the early postpartum and in terms of concern about maternal mortality at six to eight months postpartum. There was a clear stage of re-definition of 'self', not as women or as mothers but as older mothers, and this tendency was found among the majority of participants, irrespective of career investment. As such, it represents one of the few common findings among the dream-come-true and career women of this study. Interestingly, a resolution of sorts was ultimately reached by participants at approximately six months postpartum. At this stage, maternal age was reframed favourably, as contributing positively to child raising. Participants described feeling that advanced maturity and maternal characteristics such as greater patience and satisfaction with life events had contributed to greater maternal adaptation and contentment. This reframing of maternity as older maternity is a new contribution to the field and was an unanticipated finding of the current study. In addition to a reframing of maternal age, participants in this study described a re-negotiation of work and life goals as mothering assumed an unanticipated centrality in their lives, as follows.

Work and balance / confusing social messages

Confusing social messages around work and mothering were frequently discussed by study participants as contributing to maternal angst and this trend was seen almost exclusively among career women. Earlier expectations of mothering as an adjunct to the mother's work life were later replaced by an understanding of mothering as a life transforming and central event. In this study, an unanticipated depth of feeling for the infant was described by most mothers, which in turn gave rise to a revision of work plans and a re-negotiation of values as mothers came to understand mothering as the 'most important thing' in their lives. In the light of new maternal understandings and changed priorities, particular concerns centred on finding a balance between work and family. Many mothers spoke of a social undervaluing of the maternal role and a lack of appreciation of the difficulties of juggling work and family. Although this understanding of conflicting work / maternal roles is prodigiously addressed in the literature, aspects of changing maternal priorities receive scant attention. Of the few references that have been located, an age-related association is suggested (see chapter 7).

It also seems likely that, for the older professional mothers of this study, participation in the public sphere at levels of some seniority and for a considerable length of time may have contributed to an intensity of angst and struggle in the early days of mothering. In general, older professional mothers seem especially receptive to social discourses that dictate that a woman should work but also that an infant should receive almost exclusive maternal care. The reasons why this is so are not entirely clear. It may, in part, relate to a tendency to try to 'do things properly', and also to a lesser support network and fewer opportunities to view firsthand what other mothers really do. Extensive reading on the part of this group of women may also compound the dilemma, in terms of increased awareness of social expectations of the mothering role. Together, these factors impact significantly on maternal experience for primiparae over 35. However, despite common understandings of older primiparae as super-anxious and prone to high levels of postnatal depression, the women of this study were found to be proactive seekers of services and advice.

Resourceful and proactive

Here, participants did not demonstrate high levels of post-natal maladjustment as commonly associated with this group of mothers. Indeed, of the 22 older mothers in this study, only one suffered from a minor degree of postnatal depression, which is significantly less than the estimated national incidence of approximately 10-20% depression postulated for all mothers. As we shall see in a later section of this chapter, common understandings of higher incidence of postnatal depression among this group may actually relate to the high memorability of individual cases rather than to incidence alone. Close attention to the literature does not support the notion of age-related greater incidence of postnatal depression, but instead reveals that mothering over 35 years is associated with more nurturing behaviour. However, there is a concomitant understanding of this group of mothers as disadvantaged and unsupported. The findings of this study found the converse to be the case. Although many mothers identified a need for additional professional and social support initially, most were confident and pro-active in seeking assistance to meet their needs.

Additionally, though it could be argued that social context impacts meaningfully on all human experience, for primiparae over 35 the relationship between social positioning of women and maternal experience seems especially significant. A discrepancy between discourses and expectations of motherhood versus discourses of womanhood seem to adversely affect the early mothering experiences of this group of mothers, as follows.

The social context of first mothering over 35

The social context of first mothering for women over 35 has, until this point, received scant attention within the literature, despite social trends of changing female employment and later childbearing. As we have seen in chapter 2, through the medium of three women's stories, maternal experience reflects temporal social values and takes on different meanings in different historical eras. Changes over the past fifty years include trends of higher female education and greater participation in the workforce, particularly highly-paying competitive employment. These trends have contributed to a changing social emphasis on 'what is important' in the lives of modern women. A shift towards female selfhood has also given rise to expectations that women should work and compete in the public sphere and, importantly, that women may also harbour personal ambitions. This selfhood, as we saw in chapter 5, in turn gave rise to issues of self and identity as mothers struggled to position themselves within self-sacrificing models of mothering. Despite considerable change to women's life trajectories, changing discourses of womanhood appear not to have been accompanied by any lessening of maternal role expectations and the potential for conflict between women's personal ambitions and domestic roles is great. Indeed, it would seem that maternal responsibilities have expanded at a time when women have less free time than ever before. Additionally, despite apparent strong social approval for maternity, mothering does not attract the same social status as work within the public sphere, which further adds to the conundrum for women raised to value competition and individuality.

In general, there are three main messages within contemporary maternal discourses that seem to target women over 30, but especially over 35 years. Those messages are: you can do it all, meaning full-time work and mothering; you should have a baby as a social responsibility and, thirdly, mothering is an experience not to be missed. Mothers in this study discussed these social expectations as impacting negatively on their early mothering experiences. In retrospect, many described mothering expectations as both incongruent and impossible to meet. Prior to birth, participants, particularly career women, expressed a belief that good time management was the key to successful work / mothering relations and these women mostly considered that it was possible to do both well. For women who mothered in the context of career commitment, most also believed that mothering would be an adjunct to their work lives. Indeed, within discourses of working women, these views are common and mothering is portrayed as a secondary role. The second social message contributing to the quandary is the suggestion of 'doing one's duty' and 'lifting the birth-rate' that seem to be aimed principally at women over 30 (Cica, 2002). Public scrutiny of non-mothering choices among these women is also common. Choosing

217

to delay childbearing whilst pursuing career / personal ambition is regularly portrayed as selfish and aberrant (Kaplan, 1992) and women are exhorted to avail of dwindling opportunities to child bear. Consequently, the experience of maternity is often invested with a sense of urgency for women over 35, which relates to concerns over declining fertility.

In this already contested field, there is a third competing strand and mothering is depicted in glowing and eloquent terms, as a rewarding and fulfilling experience for women and as something a woman might later regret should she not avail of the opportunity. Common sources of pregnancy / mothering literature present a fragmented and sentimental picture to women anticipating motherhood. Within this view, becoming a mother is portrayed as a wonderful time. However, this incomplete picture often results in a disjuncture as expectations and experiences of mothering differ greatly. In this study, some mothers expressed a sense of having been cheated by the social mores and expectations surrounding motherhood, particularly relating to the possibility of 'doing it all' effortlessly. Whilst happy with their mothering roles and loving their infants, these women felt burdened by social expectations and limited acknowledgement of the difficulties they faced balancing work / maternal responsibilities.

Within contemporary discourse, mothering is also depicted as 'natural' and, other than some initial adjustment, easy. These discourses suggest that women who do not find mothering 'natural or easy' are themselves unnatural and this expectation places an enormous burden on contemporary women to perform well as mothers. It also limits women's opportunities for complaint or discussion when mothering is different than anticipated. Indeed, only when a woman becomes a mother is she exposed to the day-to-day realities of the role, and many women in this study spoke of a 'conspiracy' of silence around 'what mothering is really like'. Older primiparae who tend to mother in isolation seem especially susceptible to these mixed social messages.

Furthermore, a strange paradox surrounds first mothering over 35 years, particularly for professional women. On the one hand these women are portrayed as educated and knowing, making demands on doctors and health care professionals, such as caesarean section on demand (Teutsch, 2002). On the other hand, midwives and health professionals identify these mothers as vulnerable and uncertain whilst at the same time acknowledging their assertiveness.

In sum, conflicting sets of expectations create a burdensome conundrum for mothers of all ages in advanced industrial nations, such as Australia, though this experience seems to be particularly intense for primiparae over 35, who tend to mother in isolation and for whom the experience of mothering is often invested with a sense of urgency. Congruent with the discussion of the social context of older first

218

mothering, an exploration of the study's contribution to the intellectual debate surrounding this phenomenon follows.

Contribution to the intellectual debate

A post-structuralist approach has been used in this study to access the powerful though largely invisible social discourses surrounding older primiparity in a bid to expose the underlying structures for critique. In this way, an opportunity has presented for 'taken for granted' discourses to be accessed and challenged, leading the way for an examination of beliefs underpinning first mothering over 35 years. Here, participants identified struggles relating to competing and conflicting expectations around self versus baby versus work and these issues are closely paralleled within the competing discourses outlined above. In exposing these discourses, this work contributes to the intellectual debate surrounding the socio-political context of mothering, particularly as it affects first-time mothers over 35 years.

This examination of the experiences of primiparae over 35 has demonstrated the angst- inducing character of first maternity for these women and also the social constraints that conspire to silence such women as they struggle through the misery, isolation and fatigue of early mothering. As participants in this study gained understanding of their new role they came to realise that there was 'no one right way' to be a mother despite social understandings to the contrary. From that understanding, mothers moved forward to 'finding my own way', realising that in so doing they were not neglecting their infants. In retrospect, many participants here were highly critical of the constraints imposed by social expectations of mothering. These women recommended measures to dilute the powerful social messages they had absorbed. One measure suggested was the provision of more positive information on mature mothering, which is discussed in the following section of this chapter.

While it is clear that the mothers of this study were not information poor, it was also clear that there was frequently a mismatch between the information accessed by the mothers and that required. In a bid to understand the retrospectively identified needs of this group of mothers, mothers were asked at six to eight months postpartum what, if anything, midwives and health professionals could have done to better assist their transition to motherhood. In the following section feedback from the participants is presented.

Feedback from participants

This question 'what might have helped' unleashed a torrent of suggestions from study participants, which are discussed here in order of frequency of reporting. Three main areas were identified, and relate to provision of information on the 'little things' concerning the daily care of an infant, the timing of information delivery and, thirdly, the provision of more positive information about mature mothering. A brief overview of participant suggestions is attended here as a prelude to a more detailed discussion under nursing implications.

The 'little things'

Most participants here identified a distressing lack of information related to daily care of the infant, particularly recognising the tired infant, recognising the underfed infant, dealing with an ill baby, dressing the infant appropriately for the weather and, finally, caring for oneself as a mother. Recognition of the tired infant and settling the infant to sleep were identified by most mothers as particular areas of concern. As discussed in chapter 6, several mothers resorted to attending sleep clinics and schools, in a bid to 'teach' their infants to sleep and were amazed to discover that the infant behaviours they had variously interpreted as grumpiness, hunger and boredom, actually related to infant fatigue. Most felt that had they been in possession of basic information about signs of tiredness in the infant, then perhaps their experiences of an unsettled infant might have been different.

Many mothers also worried considerably about the infant getting enough food and seemed at a loss to know if the breastfed infant, in particular, was sufficiently fed. An inability to tell *exactly* how much milk the infant had imbibed was a source of concern.

Recognising the ill baby was also a continuing source of angst and many mothers worried extravagantly that the unsettled infant was unwell. It was only after the infant had had a minor illness, such as a cold, that the mother realised how an unwell infant presented. Concerns about overheating the infant were commonly voiced, particularly in relation to SIDS, and many mothers would have liked clear specific guidelines as to what constituted appropriate clothing and bedding, as discussed in chapter 6. Finally, several mothers mentioned that the first few weeks of mothering were so busy and fraught with worry that they rested very little, to their later detriment. These women would have liked information on the importance of maternal rest and recovery, particularly after caesarean section. Generally speaking, most mothers felt that the provision of a small guidebook addressing basic needs would have been useful, and further discussed many parenting guidebooks as impossibly detailed and anxiety provoking. Timing of information delivery was also discussed by a considerable percentage of the participants and is considered in the following section.

Timing of information / impossible to be fully prepared
Many mothers in this study felt inadequately prepared for going home from hospital and expressed the belief that such preparation could have been better attended both at pre-natal classes and prior to hospital discharge. Timing of information delivery was frequently discussed and, despite common beliefs to the contrary, many mothers felt they would have been receptive to infant care information delivered during pre-natal education classes or in the early postpartum period. There was also a general acknowledgment that it was impossible to be fully prepared, which is similar to suggestions raised in the literature (Barclay et al., 1997; McVeigh, 1997b).

More positive information about mature mothers
Here, many mothers felt that more positive information about mature mothering might have been helpful. These women described receiving information outlining age-related pregnancy risk, fetal disorders and age-related odds of successful fertility treatment. Most suggested that they perhaps were not so much empowered by having this information, as terrified by the burden such knowledge imposed. Knowing that 'it would get easier' might also have made a difference to the experiences of the older mothers, again particularly career women. Several felt that understanding that things would ultimately improve might have given them the strength to carry on, when early mothering proved to be exhausting and difficult. In the following section, implications for nursing and midwifery practice are discussed, as informed by the study's findings and participant feedback.

Implications for nursing / midwifery practice

> *"I think it's about making them feel comfortable, so if they do have a difficulty they can approach you"*
>
> (Deirdre, M&CHN)

As we have seen in this study, primiparae over 35 have concerns and educational needs that differ from those expressed by younger mothers and it is important to raise awareness of the needs and anxieties of this group of women. Specifically, it is essential that we, as midwives and nurses, challenge the perception of high-risk pregnancy in this healthy cohort. There is a real need to dispel common misconceptions of maladjustment and postnatal depression, as these impressions seem to influence the subsequent care mothers receive. In highlighting the concerns expressed by the studied mothers and their particular difficulties around losing face when seeking information from health professionals, it is hoped that health professionals may challenge existing practices and perceptions of the older mother and seek ways to provide these women with the information and assistance they require. Understanding that primiparae over 35 approach motherhood in a different than standard way, but ultimately are confident and resourceful in obtaining requisite information and services, may help de-bunk common conceptions of this group of women as 'hopeless'.

In the following section a series of recommendations for practice are dealt with in sequence. Those recommendations include campaigning to have care of the mother over 35 included on midwifery curricula; strategies to formalise existing casual care arrangements, maintaining efforts to dispel common misconceptions of maladjustment and postnatal depression, raising awareness of the health of this cohort in terms of risk status and diminution of the levels of anxiety. Finally, recommendations for further research are advised.

Campaigning to include first-time mothers over 35 on midwifery curricula

It is my contention that care of the first-time mother over 35 years should be included on the curricula for student midwives and updates for registered midwives and other health professionals, just as cultural and religious issues are included. Such provision may raise awareness of the vulnerability of this group and ultimately affect the way in which these women's needs are met. For example, this study found that participants would often pretend they were managing well, rather than ask for assistance, particularly if the 'vibes' from the midwife or carer were unfavourable. These women particularly valued respectful engagement and many described disliking to be patronised, spoken down to, or 'told off' by nursing staff. In possession of this knowledge, midwives and other health professionals might approach the woman differently, effectively offering her an opportunity to ask what she might consider to be 'dumb' questions. While it is clear that all new mothers would benefit from empathetic and sensitive care, older mothers in this study identified a particular need for confidence building in the early days of mothering. Similar to Pridham et al.'s, (1991) exhortation that "nurses should assess the sense of capability of more highly educated mothers and provide support that increases confidence in the knowledge and skills that they have" (p. 29), I would suggest that encouraging the mother to believe that she 'could do it' and providing sensitive care with clear simple instructions, while at the same time leaving the way open for her to ask additional questions, would considerably assist her in gaining confidence in her mothering abilities.

Strategies to formalise existing casual care arrangements

As discussed in chapter 7, midwives and M&CHNs in this study present a consensus of opinion that older primiparae generally, though not exclusively, require an additional day in hospital and additional public health visits. Consistent findings in this study indicate that these women are often ill prepared at time of discharge from hospital. On-going difficulties with establishing lactation also present. Nurses and midwives here regularly instituted differing care regimes to accommodate the commonly understood additional needs of this group of women. These differing regimes involved negotiating with hospital administration for additional hospital time and casual arrangements to provide more nursing time, invitations to the mothers to 'pop in' to health centres or to phone or visit the maternity unit for advice and/or assistance. Findings of this study suggest that although these women are not significantly at greater risk than younger counterparts, they tend to require more nursing time and resources. Requirements of additional assistance with breastfeeding and 'ordinary' care of the infant, as identified by midwives and M&CHNs, are closely aligned to concerns and suggestions raised by the mothers of this study.

Casual nursing arrangements, as described by the midwives and M&CHNs in this study, are unsustainable in the long term, particularly as the numbers of older primiparae continue to grow. Several measures that would contribute to an improvement of care for these women are suggested here. Those suggestions include the routine allocation of a different health care coding to primigravidae over 35, as a higher-needs category, which could result in the routine allocation of an additional day in hospital and/or additional community support. Although financial constraints limit the possibility of a universal adoption of such a policy, private health insurance companies may be willing to consider covering this additional cost, knowing that it may positively effect future care requirements such as admission to mother and baby units or sleep centres. Secondly, additional pre-natal and neonatal classes aimed at meeting the needs identified by the women could be instituted at the care facility where the mothers give birth, in a bid to better equip the mothers for discharge. Although the targeted audience would be the older primiparae, such classes should be available for all new mothers. Finally, the provision of clear specific information in the form of a booklet, as discussed in a later section of this chapter, is posited.

Dispelling the myths

One of the most surprising findings of this study was, for me, understanding that primiparae over 35 are not particularly represented in postnatal depression statistics, as is commonly believed by doctors, midwives and maternal and child health nurses. A review of the literature around older maternity, in fact, supports the converse view and maternal maturity appears to augur well for maternal adjustment. Similarly to my colleagues, I too, had thought that postnatal depression and maladjustment were more commonly seen in this group, though I was confused by the paradox this situation offered. Impressions of increased prevalence of postnatal depression are very common misrepresentations and may stem, in part, from the fact that midwives and obstetricians who care for these women, principally do so around the peri-natal period, when the older primipara is at her 'worst'. This may, in effect, inform the skewed perception of poorer maternal adaptation that health professionals hold.

Interestingly, when I spoke to a variety of health professionals in a bid to understand how this myth of poorer maternal adjustment had become so prevalent, the almost invariable response was that these women were particularly prone to depression and this was presented as an unquestionable fact. When I asked one obstetrician how many depressed older mothers he had seen in his practice in the last ten years, both he and I were surprised to realise he could remember and name each of the older professional mothers he had referred elsewhere for care of their depression. His exclamation that they were so much trouble that one would never forget them, made me think of what my supervisor calls the one equals ten rule, that one woman of this ilk suffering from postnatal depression or extreme anxiety, was as much trouble, in terms of phone calls and visits, as ten standard women. Similarly, among the midwives and M&CHNs, most could name one or two professional older mothers who had significant postnatal distress or depression and were surprised to find that the numbers were actually quite small. This situation of high memorability may in turn contribute to an inflated impression of occurrence.

Raising awareness in terms of 'risk status'

It is important to challenge existing perceptions of age alone as a predictor of pregnancy risk status among older mothers, for being considered 'at risk' undoubtedly increases maternal angst and worry. Generally speaking, first-time mothers over 35 tend to be well-educated and financially secure and, as such, they are likely to pursue healthy lifestyle choices and to abstain from smoking. Higher maternal education also results in increased health awareness and better access to health care. Risks for this healthy and well-educated group are likely to be significantly less than for older mothers of 20-30 years ago, who tended to be associated with socio-economic disadvantage. Despite marked socio-

224

demographic changes, much of the medical literature relating to older mothering is informed by an earlier group of older mothers and perceptions of age-related increased risk still prevail. To date, medical research has focused primarily on the complications of older childbearing, such as increased incidence of high blood pressure and gestational diabetes but has not generally addressed lifestyle influences, such as smoking, weight and general health. Further research is needed to identify the real risks of advanced maternal age among healthy older primiparae. Nurses and midwives need to challenge the perception of high-risk pregnancy for these women. A less high-risk approach to pregnancy may reduce the anxiety that many older mothers feel. These well-informed, healthy women can then become more involved in their care in collaboration with their nurse or midwife.

Diminution of the levels of anxiety

In order to diminish the anxiety levels suffered by a considerable percentage of primiparae over 35 and in line with the needs identified by the mothers of this study, the following simple measures are proposed: adoption of efforts to normalise the experience of pregnancy and birth for these women; provision of written information around identified areas of concern.

Normalising the experience

Nursing and midwifery emphasis should be on de-mystifying and normalising the process of childbearing for this group of women, many of whom consider their pregnancy and birth to be an exceptional event (a miracle). Constant reminders that the infant is a 'little person' and thus has bodily needs similar to their own, for example, food and warmth, may help ground the experience of childbearing within the realm of 'normal'. Provision of concrete examples may also help dispel disproportionate fears and figures should be presented in a realistic manner. For example, a SIDS risk of 1:1,000, may mean that in 15-20 years of being a M&CHN or midwife and caring for hundreds of mothers and infants, that one sees only one or perhaps no infant succumb to SIDS, which may make the risk seem considerably less than the term 'leading cause of death' suggests.

Understanding too that this may be the first real experience the mother has ever had of holding an infant, or having anything more than a cursory glance to do with a small child, may help the midwife or carer to locate the woman's experience and to realise that 'taken for granted' meanings, known by every midwife, are not necessarily known by the new mother. For example, explaining that the infant's refusal at the breast is more likely related to poor milk flow, or positioning of the newborn's painful bruised head, may lessen the likelihood that the mother feels rejected by her baby. Similarly, removing

225

the baby to give Mum a break, although meant kindly, may intensify the women's sense of failure and helplessness, unless accompanied by a reasonable explanation. What may work considerably better is to settle the baby in the mother's presence, explaining how it was achieved, or coach the mother through settling techniques.

Provision of written information around identified areas of concern:

In this study, there was a tendency among the mothers to require clear specific guidelines on everyday infant care and the absence of such instruction made the initial days of mothering very uncertain. Such information should address simple signs of fatigue such as rubbing the eyes, or grizzling, which were often misinterpreted by the mothers of this study. A clear guideline of infant feeding requirements should also be included, with concrete examples of how to assess the infant's sufficient intake. Suggesting perhaps that the infant should have six wet nappies[*] in twenty-four hours may help the concerned mother assess the sufficiency of intake. Clear guidelines on recognising the ill infant may also help dispel disproportionate concerns regarding the infant's health. Knowing that the unwell infant might be listless and disinterested in feeding might have helped allay the daily anxieties suffered by some mothers. Similarly, the provision of simple guidelines on dressing the infant, for example, to dress the infant in similar weight clothing as the mother but with the addition of an extra layer or blanket / wrap may make dressing the infant appropriately less onerous. Finally, steering the women away from medicalised information may be helpful, as most study participants felt that such information fuelled rather than alleviated anxiety. However, in practice, this may be difficult to achieve, as mothers in this study suggested that denial of access to requested information may have fuelled their anxieties and information quests.

More positive feedback on the positive effects of mature mothering

The provision of positive information relating to mature mothering was often raised by the mothers of this study. Many mothers described an inability to find age-related literature other than that concentrating on the medical risks of advanced maternal age and associated increased rates of chromosomal abnormality. Positive information was difficult to obtain and most felt they would have benefited from knowing that it was 'not all bad news.' To that end, information for mothers, highlighting the fact that infants of mothers over 35 fare little differently than the infants of younger

---

[*] Diapers

mothers, in terms of mortality and morbidity, could be made available to this group of mothers. This knowledge may help reduce maternal concerns and perceptions of vulnerability in the infant.

Until this point the discussion has centred on the study findings and possible recommendations for care. Now it is important to discuss the strengths and limitations of the study and to make recommendations for further research.

Limitations / strengths of the study / recommendations for research

In this study, findings are restricted by the small sample size and some limitations of sample variety are also acknowledged. In particular, the inclusion criteria has excluded several groups of women, for example, non-English speaking women and women choosing to give birth in alternate locations, such as home births. The voice of primiparae over 35 years from lower socio-economic groupings is also poorly represented, despite inclusion efforts. Participants in this study mostly represented well-educated middle-class mothers, and interpretations of the findings of this study must therefore be restricted to this population. There is additionally a concern that the mothers choosing to give birth at the tertiary hospital where participants were recruited may represent a particular group of women who may perhaps be prone to exaggerated concerns.

However, the longitudinal nature of the study facilitated opportunities for clarification of intent and later pursuit of interesting / unanticipated information arising from the data. This 'second chance' is recognised here as a methodological strength. It could also be argued that the homogeneity of the sample may add to the likelihood of greater insight into the experiences of mothering over 35 for this particular group of mothers, by offering an opportunity to access multiple accounts. Finally, participants in this study appear to represent current demographic trends of higher maternal education and career investment among older first-time mothers.

Although the findings of this study are both limited and tentative, they give rise to some interesting questions for further research. For example: what effect, if any, does socio-economic status and high educational level have on mothering over 35? Do the findings discovered here apply only to first mothering? How is second or subsequent mothering experienced by mothers over 35 years? Although the intent of this study was an examination of first mothering over 35, the question 'How does the experience of first fathering affect men aged over 35 years?' presents as an interesting area for additional study.

Overall, the general paucity of qualitative research literature into first mothering over 35 years is striking and efforts to address this dearth should be encouraged. Specifically, professional women with significant career investment seem to present as a distinct cohort and merit further qualitative research endeavour. Large-scale quantitative studies are also necessary to address the 'real' risks of advanced maternal age in a healthy population. Such research has the potential to extend the body of medical literature and go some way towards establishing or refuting current ideas of age-related maternal risk.

Summary

In conclusion, changing social trends mean that Australia, like other developed countries, will continue to see increasing numbers of childbearing women aged over 35 and a considerable portion of this group will be first-time mothers. At the same time, dwindling health resources will continue to reduce maternal services, with possible major implications for the health of the older mother and her infant. It is therefore imperative that health care professionals learn as much as possible about the specific needs of this group of healthy women, who appear to experience considerable distress and disproportionate concern for the infant during their transition to motherhood. Simple measures such as providing clear specific guidelines for infant care may go some way towards addressing the needs and anxieties of this group, as may attempts to de-mystify and normalise the experience of pregnancy for these women.

Another significant area of concern is the perpetuation of inaccurate beliefs of mothering over 35 as associated with higher than average levels of postnatal depression and maladjustment. There is a clearly identified need for further qualitative endeavour to explicate the experiences of first-time mothers over 35, particularly those women who have electively delayed childbearing, while pursuing career and personal ambitions. These women present as a distinct cohort, with concerns and needs that differ from other new mothers. Further medical research is also suggested in a bid to establish the 'real' risks of advanced maternal age in a healthy cohort.

The significance of the current study rests in the contribution it makes to the intellectual debate surrounding the social context of delayed childbearing. The contribution it makes to nursing literature is also significant and this work and the papers published from the study have added considerably to the scant body of literature addressing first mothering over 35 years. Finally, in identifying the specific needs of this group, health professionals may be enabled to provide more meaningful maternal support and to more effectively promote maternal well-being among this growing group of mothers.

References

Abrams, L. R., & Jones, R.W. (1997). *The contribution of social roles to psychological distress in businesswomen.* Melbourne, Australia: University of Melbourne, Department of Science and Mathematics.

Ainsworth, M. D., Yarrow, L. J., & Glaser, K. (1962). *Maternal deprivation.* New York: Child Welfare League of America.

Aldous, M. B., & Edmonson, M. B. (1993). Maternal age at first childbirth and risk of low birth weight and pre-term delivery in Washington State, *Journal of the American Medical Association, 270*(21), 2574-2577.

Altheide, D. E., & Johnson, J. M. (1994). Criteria for assessing interpretative validity in qualitative research. In N. Denzin & Y. Lincoln (Eds.), *Handbook of qualitative research* (pp. 485-499). London: Sage.

Alvarez, L. (2003). Norway leads industrial nations back to breastfeeding. *New York Times*, p. 3.

Alvesson, M., & Skoldberg, K. (2000). *Reflexive methodology.* London: Sage.

Ambler Walter, C. (1986). *The timing of motherhood.* Massachusetts: Lexington.

Anderson, A. M. N., Wohlfahrt, J., Christens, P., Olsen, J., & Melbye, M. (2000). Maternal age and fetal loss: Population based register linkage study. *British Medical Journal, 320*, 1708-1712.

Andrews, M., Lyne, P., & Riley, E. (1996). Validity in qualitative healthcare research: An exploration of the impact of individual researcher perspectives within collaborative inquiry. *Journal of Advanced Nursing, 23*(3), 441-447.

Antonucci, T. C., & Mikus, K. (1988). The power of parenthood: Personality and attitudinal changes during the transition to parenthood. In G. Y. Michaels & W. A. Goldberg (Eds.), *Transition to parenthood: Current theory and research* (pp. 62-84). New York: Cambridge University Press.

Appleton, J. V. (1995). Analysing qualitative interview data: Addressing issues of validity and reliability. *Journal of Advanced Nursing, 22*(5), 993-997.

Apter, T. E. (1993). *Professional progress: Why women still don't have wives.* London: Macmillan.

Arndt, B. (2002, September 10). Do political mums really know best? Melbourne: *The Age*, p. 10.

Auerbach, K. (1990). Assisting the employed breastfeeding mother. *Journal of Nurse Midwifery, 35*(1), 26-34.

Australian Bureau of Statistics (1995). *National health survey: Private health insurance (ABS publication no. 4334.0)*. Canberra: Australian Government Press.

Australian Bureau of Statistics (2000). *Births, Australia 1999 (ABS publication no. 3301)*. Canberra: Australian Government Press.

Australian Bureau of Statistics (2003a). *Births, Australia 2002 (ABS publication no. 3301.0)*. Canberra: Australian Government Press.

Australian Bureau of Statistics (2003b). *Breastfeeding in Australia (ABS publication no. 4810.0.55.001)*. Canberra: Australian Government Press.

Australian Institute of Health and Welfare, National Perinatal Statistics Unit (2000). *Catalogue no. PER15*. Canberra: Australian Government Press.

Badinter, E. (1981). *The Motherhood myth: an historical view of the maternal instinct.* London: Souvenir.

Bagwell, J., Kendrick, O. W., Stitt, K. R., Leeper, J. D., Espy, M. L., & Gedel, M. L. (1992). Breastfeeding among women in the Alabama WIC Program. *Journal of Human Lactation* 8(4), 205-8.

Baiagioli, F. (2003). Returning to work while breastfeeding. *American Family Physician* 68(11), 2201-2208.

Bailey, P., & Tilley, S. (2002). Storytelling and the interpretation of meaning in qualitative research. *Journal of Advanced Nursing*, 38(6), 574-583.

Baltes, P. B. (1987). Theoretical propositions of life span developmental psychology: On the dynamics between growth and decline. *Developmental Psychology*, 23, 611-626.

Barclay, L., & Lloyd, B. (1996). The misery of motherhood: Alternate approaches to maternal distress. *Midwifery*, 12, 136-139.

Barclay, L., Everitt, L., Rogan, F., Schmied, V., & Wyllie, A. (1997). Becoming a mother: An analysis of women's experiences of early motherhood. *Journal of Advanced Nursing*, 25(4), 719-728.

Barkan, S. E., & Bracken, M. B. (1987)[*]. Delayed childbearing: No evidence for increased risk of low birth weight and pre-term delivery. *American Journal of Epidemiology*, 125, 101-109.

Barlow, C. A., & Cairns, K. V. (1997). Mothering as a psychological experience: A grounded theory exploration. *Canadian Journal of Counselling*, 31(3), 232-247.

Barton, J. R., Bergauer, N. K., Jacques, D. L., Coleman, S. K., Stanziano, G. J., & Sibai, B. M. (1997). Does advanced maternal age affect pregnancy outcome in women with mild hypertension remote from term? *American Journal of Obstetrics and Gynecology*, 176, 1236-43.

---

[*] footnote reference

Belsky, J., Ward, M. J., & Rovine, M. (1986). Prenatal expectations, postnatal experiences and the transition to parenthood. In R. Ashmore & D. Brodzinsky (Eds.), *Thinking about the family: Views of parents and children* (pp.119-145). Hillsdale NJ: Lawrence Erlbaum.

Benn, M. (1998). *Madonna and child: Towards a new politics of motherhood.* London, Jonathan Cape.

Bennett, V. R., & Brown, L. K. (1999). *Myles textbook for midwives.* Edinburgh: Churchill Livingstone.

Bergum, V. (1989). *Woman to mother: A transformation.* Massachussetts: Bergin & Garvey.

Bergum, V. (1997). *A child on her mind: The experience of becoming a woman.* Westport, Connecticut: Bergin & Garvey.

Berkowitz, G. S., Shovron, M. L., Lapinski, R. H., & Berkowitz, R. L. (1993). Does delayed childbearing increase risk? *Journal of the American Medical Association,* 269, 745-748.

Berryman, J. C. (1991). Perspectives on later motherhood. In A. Phoenix, A. Woollett & E. Lloyd (Eds.), *Motherhood, meanings, practices and ideologies* (pp. 103- 122). London: Sage.

Berryman, J. C., Thorpe, K., & Windridge, K. C. (1999). *Older mothers, conception, pregnancy and birth after 35.* London: Harper Collins.

Berryman, J. C., & Windridge, K. C. (1995). *Motherhood after 35: A report on the Leicester motherhood project.* Leicester: Leicester University.

Berryman, J. C., & Windridge, K. C. (1996). Pregnancy after 35 and attachment to the fetus. *Journal of Reproductive and Infant Psychology,* 14, 133-143.

Bewley, C. (1999). Postnatal depression. *Nursing Standard,* 13, 49-56.

232

Bobrowski, R. A., & Bottoms, S. F. (1995). Underappreciated risks of the elderly multipara. *American Journal of Obstetrics and Gynecology,* 172, 1764-70.

Bonellie, S. R. (2001). Effect of maternal age, smoking and deprivation on birthweight. *Paediatric and Perinatal Epidemiology,* 15, 19-26.

Borjesson, B., Paperin, C., & Lindell, M. (2004). Maternal support during the first year of infancy. *Journal of Advanced Nursing,* 45(6), 588-594.

Bowlby, J. (1953). *Child care and the growth of love.* Middlesex UK: Penguin.

Bowling, A. (2002). *Research methods in health: investigating health and health services.* Philadelphia, Open University Press.

Brannen, J., & Moss, P. (1991). *Managing mothers: Dual earning households after maternity leave.* London: Unwin Hyman.

Brazelton, T. B. (1992). *Touchpoints: The essential reference guide to your child's emotional and behavioural development.* Sydney: Doubleday.

Brazelton, T. B., & Sparrow, J.A. (2001). *Touchpoints 3-6: understanding your child's emotional and behavioural development.* Oxford: Perseus.

Brodribb, W. (1992). *Breastfeeding and breast surgery.* (Topics in Breastfeeding, set iv). Melbourne, Australia: Lactation Resource Centre.

Brodribb, W. (1997). *Breastfeeding management in Australia* (2nd ed) Melbourne: Nursing Mothers Association Australia.

Brown, S., Lumley, J., Small, R., & Astbury, J. (1994). *Missing voices: The experience of motherhood.* Melbourne, Australia: Oxford University Press.

233

Bruner, J. (1984). Introduction: The opening up of anthropology. In S. Plattner & E. M. Bruner (Eds.), *Text, play and story: The construction and reconstruction of self and society* (pp. 1-16). Washington DC: American Ethnological Society.

Bruner, J. (1986). *Actual minds, possible words*. London: Harvard University Press.

Bryman, A. (2001). *Social research methods*. New York, Oxford University Press.

Burkett, E. (2000). *The baby boon: How family-friendly America cheats the childless*. New York: Free Press.

Burr, W. R., Leigh, G. K., Day, R. D., & Constandine, J. (1979). Symbolic interaction and the family. In W.R. Burr, R. Hill, F. I. Nye & I. L. Reiss (Eds.), *Contemporary theories about the family* (Vol. 2, pp. 42-111). New York: Free Press.

Burrage, J. (1998). Infertility treatment in women aged over 40 years. *Nursing Standard,* 13(5), 43-45.

Butler, J. (1990). *Gender trouble: Feminism and the subversion of identity*. New York: Routledge.

Butler, J. (1992). *Feminists theorize the political*. New York, Routledge.

Butler, J. (1996). From the subversion of identity to the subversion of solidarity? *Sacrificial logics: feminist theory and the critique of identity.* A. Weir. London, Routledge: 112-134.

Carolan, M. C. (2003a). Reflexivity: A personal journey through data collection. *Nurse Researcher,* 10(3), 7-14.

Carolan, M. C. (2003b). The graying of the obstetric population: Implications for the older mother. *Journal of Obstetric, Gynecologic, and Neonatal Nursing*, 32(1), 19-27.

Carolan, M. C. (2003c). Later motherhood: The experience of parturition for first-time mothers aged >35 years. *Australian Midwifery*, 16(2), 17-21.

Carolan, M. C. (2004). Women's narratives of early mothering: Getting past the 'right story'. *Birth Issues, 13*(2), 51-56.

Carolan, M. C. (in press-a). The role of stories in understanding life events: Post-structural construction of the 'self'. *Collegian.*

Carolan, M. C. (in press-b). Maternal and child health nurses: A vital link to the community for primiparae over the age of 35. *Contemporary Nurse.*

Carolan, M. C. (in press-c). Anxiety in primiparous mothers > 35: Challenges for care? *Birth Issues.*

Cavanagh, S. (1997). Content analysis: concepts, methods and applications. *Nurse Researcher* 4(3), 5-16.

Chase, S. E. (1995). *Ambiguous empowerment: The work narratives of women school superintendents.* Amherst: University of Massachusetts Press.

Chesney, M. (2000). Interaction and understanding 'me' in the research. *Nurse Researcher, 7*(3), 58-69.
Chezem, J., Friesen, C., & Boettcher, J. (2003). Breastfeeding knowledge, breastfeeding confidence, and infant feeding plans: Effects on actual feeding practices. *Journal of Obstetric, Gynecologic, and Neonatal Nursing, 32*(1), 40-47.

Chick, N., & Meleis, A. I. (1986). Transitions: A nursing concern. In P. L. Chinn (Ed.), *Nursing research methodology: Issues and implementation* (pp. 237-257). Rockville, Maryland: Aspen.

Cica, N. (2002, August 26). 30-something women of Australia: We can repel the witch-hunt. Melbourne: *The Age*, p. 11.

Cliff, D., & Deery, R. (1997). Too much like school: Social class, age, marital status and attendance / non-attendance at pre-natal classes. *Midwifery,* 13, 139-145.

Clifford, C. (1997). *Qualitative research methodology in nursing and health care*. New York, Churchill Livingstone.

Cnattingius, S., Forman, M. R., Berendes, H. W., & Isotalo, L. (1992). Delayed childbearing and risk of adverse perinatal outcome. *Journal of the American Medical Association, 268,* 886.

Cohen, M. A., & Sauer, M. V. (1998). Fertility in peri-menopausal women. *Clinical Obstetrics and Gynecology, 41,* 958-965.

Cohen, R. L. (1979). Maladaptation to pregnancy. *Seminars in Perinatology, 3,* 15-24.

Cooey, P. M. (1999). Ordinary mother as oxymoron. In J. E. Hanigsberg & S. Ruddick (Eds.), *Mother troubles* (pp. 229-249). Boston: Beacon Press.

Cook, C. B. (1993). Perceived psychological stress, perceived adequacy of social supports, and perceived social networks of first-time mothers 20-25 and 30-35 years of age (Doctoral dissertation, Wayne State University, 1993). *Dissertations Abstracts International, 55,* 03.

Cooke, M. (2000). Postnatal care: What do women want? *Nursing Review, 15,* (August).

Corbett-Dick, P., & Bezek, S. K. (1997). Breastfeeding promotion for the employed mother. *Journal of Pediatric Health Care, 11,* 12-19.

Cowan, P. A., & Cowan, C. P. (1995). Interventions to ease the transition to parenthood. *Family Relations, 44,* 412-423.

Coward, R. (1997). The heaven and hell of mothering: Mothering and ambivalence in the mass media. In W. Hollway & B. Featherstone (Eds.), *Mothering and ambivalence* (pp. 111-118). London: Routledge.

Crittenden, A. (2001). *The price of motherhood: Why the most important job in the world is still the least valued.* New York: Henry Holt.

Crouch, M. & Manderson, L. (1993). *New motherhood: Cultural and personal transitions in the 1980s.* Melbourne: Gordon & Breach.

Crowe, M. (1998). The power of the word: Some post-structural considerations of qualitative approaches in nursing research. *Journal of Advanced Nursing,* 28(2), 339-344.

Cudmore, L. G. (1997). The transition to motherhood: A phenomenological study of women's experiences as first-time mothers. (Doctoral dissertation, University of Ottawa, 1997). *Digital Abstracts International, 58,* 10.

Cunningham, G. F., & Leveno, K. J. (1995). Childbearing among older women: The message is cautiously optimistic. *The New England Journal of Medicine*, 333, 1002-1004.

Cutcliffe, J. (2000). Methodological issues in grounded theory. *Journal of Advanced Nursing*, 31, 1476-1484.

Cutcliffe, J., & McKenna, H. (1999). Establishing the credibility of qualitative research findings: The plot thickens. *Journal of Advanced Nursing*, 30, 374-380.

Dally, A. (1982). *Inventing motherhood: The consequences of an ideal.* London: Burnett.

Danaher, G., Schirato, T., & Webb, J. (2000). *Understanding Foucault.* St. Leonards, NSW, Australia: Allen & Unwin.

Daniels, P., & Weingarten, K. (1982). *Sooner or later: The timing of parenthood in adult lives.* New York: Norton.

Davies, B. (1991). The concept of agency: A feminist post-structuralist analysis. *Social Analysis*, 30, 42-53.

Davies, B., & Harre, R. (2001). Positioning: The discursive production of selves. In M. Wetherell, S.Taylor & S. J. Yates (Eds.), *Discourse theory and practice* (pp. 261-271). Thousand Oaks: Sage.

237

De Beauvoir, S. (1952). *The second sex.* New York: Vintage Books.

deMause, L. (1974). The evolution of childhood. In L. deMause (Ed.), *The history of childhood* (pp. 1-73). London: Souvenir Press.

Dennis, C. L., Hodnett, E., Gallop, R., & Chalmers, B. (2002). The effect of peer support on breastfeeding duration among primiparous women: A randomised controlled trial. *Canadian Medical Association Journal,* 166(1), 21-28.

Deutsch, F. M. (1999). *Halving it all: How equally shared parenting really works.* Cambridge, Massachusetts: Harvard University Press.

Deutsch, F. M., Brooks-Gunn, J., Fleming, A., Ruble, D. N., & Stangor, C. (1988). Information seeking and maternal self-definition during the transition to motherhood. *Journal of Personality and Social Psychology,* 55, 420-421.

Dildy G. A., Jackson, G. M., Fowers, G. K., Oshiro, B. T., Varner, M. W., & Clark, S. L. (1996). Very advanced maternal age: Pregnancy after age 45. *American Journal of Obstetrics and Gynecology,* 175, 668-674.

DiQuinzio, P. (1999). *The impossibility of motherhood: Feminism, individualism and the problem with mothering.* New York: Routledge.

Dobrzykowski, T. M. (1998). The spiraling process of childbirth after the age of 30: Mature mothering and no unfinished business. (Doctoral dissertation, Indiana University, 1998). *Digital Abstracts International B 59,* 02.

Dobrzykowski, T. M., & Stern, P. N. (2003). Out of sync: A generation of first-time mothers over 30. *Health Care for Women International,* 24, 242-253.

Doering, L., Moser, D. K., & Dracup K. (2000). Correlates of anxiety, hostility, depression, and psychosocial adjustment in parents of NICU infants. *Journal of Neonatal Nursing,* 19, 5, 15-23.

Downe-Wamboldt, B. (1992). Content analysis: method, applications, and issues. *Health Care for Women International* 13(3): 313-21.

Drummond, J., McBride, M. L., & Wiebe, C. F. (1993). The development of mothers' understanding of infant crying. *Clinical Nursing Research,* 2(4), 396-413.

Earland, J., Ibrahim, S. O., & Hairpin, V. A. (1997). Maternal employment: Does it influence feeding practices during infancy? *Journal of Human Nutrition and Diabetes,* 10(5), 305-311.

Easterbrooks, M. A. (1988). Effects of infant risk on the transition to parenthood. In G. Y. Michaels & W. A. Goldberg (Eds.), *Transition to parenthood: Current theory and research* (pp. 176-208). New York: Cambridge University Press.

Ehrenreich, B., & English, D. (1988). *For her own good: 150 years of the experts' advice to women.* London: Pluto Press.

Eisenstein, H. (1984). *Contemporary feminist thought.* St Leonards, New South Wales, Australia: Allen & Unwin.

Elliot, R., Drummond, J., & Barnard, K. E. (1996). Subjective appraisal of infant crying. *Clinical Nursing Research,* 5(2), 237-250.

Ellis, C., Kiesinger, C. E., & Tillmann-Healy, L. M. (1997). Interactive interviewing: Talking about emotional experience. In R. Hertz (Ed.), *Reflexivity and voice* (pp. 119-149). Thousand Oaks: Sage.

Emden, C. (1998). Conducting a narrative analysis. *Collegian*, 5(3), 34-39.

Emmanuel, E., Creedy, D., & Fraser, J. (2001). What mothers want: A postnatal survey. *Australian Midwifery,* 14(4), 16-20.

Erikson, E. (1978). *Adulthood.* New York: W.W. Norton.

239

Erlandson, D. A., Harris, E. L., Skipper, B. L., & Allen, S. D. (1993). *Doing naturalistic inquiry: A guide to methods*. London: Sage.

Erlandsson, L., & Eklund, M. (2003). Women's experiences of hassles and uplifts in their everyday patterns of occupation. *Occupational Therapy International,* 10(2), 95-114.

Eyer, D. (1996). *Motherguilt: How our culture blames mothers for what's wrong with society*. New York: Times Books.

Ezzy, D. (2002). *Qualitative analysis: Practice and innovation*. Crows Nest, N.S.W, Australia: Allen & Unwin.

Fahy, K. (1997). Postmodern feminist emancipatory research: Is it an oxymoron? *Nursing Inquiry,* 4(1), 27-33.

Falk, M. (2000). The real and ideal mother: The experience of motherhood in light of the ideal. (Doctoral dissertation, California Institute of Integral Studies, San Francisco, 2000). *Digital Abstracts International, 61,10.*

Fallows, C. (1994). *The Australian baby and childcare handbook*. Melbourne: Penguin.

Feldman, S. S., & Nash, S. C. (1986). Antecedents of early parenting. In A. Fogel & G.F. Melson (Eds.), *Origins of nurturance* (pp. 209 -232). Hillsdale NJ: Laurence Erlbaum.

Ferber, R. (1987). *Solve your child's sleep problems*. Ringwood, Victoria, Australia: Penguin.

Ferber, R. (1999). *Solve your child's sleep problems*. Sydney: Dorling Kindersley.

Ferguson, A. (1989). *Blood at the root: Motherhood, sexuality and male dominance*. London: Pandora.

Ferguson, M. (1983). *Forever feminine: Women's magazines and the cult of femininity.* London: Heinemann.

Ferketich, S. L., & Mercer, R. T. (1990). Effects of antepartal stress on health status during early motherhood. *Scholarly Inquiry for Nursing Practice,* 4(2), 127-149.

Fildes, V. A. (1990). Maternal feelings re-assessed: Child abandonment and neglect in London and Westminister, 1550- 1800. In V. A. Fildes (Ed.), *Women as mothers in pre-industrial England* (pp. 139-178). London: Routledge.

Filene, P. E. (1998). *His/ her/self: sex roles in modern America.* Baltimore: John Hopkins University Press.

Finch, J. (1999). It's great to have someone to talk to: The ethics and politics of interviewing women. In A. Bryman & R. G. Burgess (Eds.), *Qualitative research* (pp. 68-80). Thousand Oaks: Sage.

Finlay, L. (1998). Reflexivity: An essential component for all research. *British Journal of Occupational Therapy,* 61(10), 453-456.

Fisher, J., Feekery, C. J., Amir, L. H., & Sneddon, M. (2002). Health and social circumstances of women admitted to a private mother baby unit: A descriptive cohort study. *Australian Family Physician,* 31(10), 966-970.

Fleming, A. S., Flett, G. L., Ruble, D. N., & Shaul, D. L. (1988). Postpartum adjustment in first-time mothers: Relations between mood, maternal attitudes and other-infant interactions. *Developmental Psychology,* 24, 71-81.

Fontana, A., & Frey, J. H. (1998). Interviewing, the art of science. In N. K. Denzin & Y. Lincoln (Eds.), *Collecting and interpreting qualitative materials* (pp. 47-78). Thousand Oaks: Sage.

Ford, M., & Hodnett, E. (1990). Predictors of adaptation in women hospitalised during pregnancy. *Canadian Journal of Nursing Research,* 22(4), 37-50.

241

Forman, D. N., Videbech, P., Hedegaard, M., Salvig, J. D., & Secher, N. J. (2000). Postpartum depression: Identification of women at risk. *British Journal of Obstetrics and Gynaecology*, 107, 1210-1217.

Forna, A. (1998). *Mother of all myths: How society moulds and constrains mothers.* London: Harper Collins.

Foucault, M. (1980). *Power / knowledge: Selected interviews and other writings 1972-77.* New York: Pantheon.

Foucault, M. (1988a). The ethic and care of the self as a practice of freedom: An interview with Michel Foucault, January 20th 1984. In J. Bernauer & G. Rasmussen (Eds.), *The Final Foucault* (pp. 1-20). Cambridge: MIT Press.

Foucault, M. (1988b). Technologies of the self. In L. H. Martin (Ed.), *Technologies of the self: A seminar with Michel Foucault* (pp. 16-49). London: Tavistock.

Foucault, M. (1988c). Truth, power, self: An interview with Michel Foucault, October 25th 1982. In L. H. Martin (Ed.), *Technologies of the self: A seminar with Michel Foucault* (pp. 9-15). London: Tavistock.

Foucault, M. (1989). *The archaeology of knowledge* (A.M. Sheridan Smith, trans). London: Tavistock. (Original work published 1972).

Foucault, M. (1991). A question of method. In G. Burchell, C. Gordon & P. Miller (Eds.), *The Foucault effect: Studies in governmentality* (pp. 87-104). Chicago: Chicago University Press.

Frank, E. (1998). Breastfeeding and maternal employment: Two rights don't make a wrong. *Lancet*, 352(9134), 1083-1084.

Freely, M., & Pyper, C. (1993). *Pandora's clock: Understanding our fertility.* London: Heinemann.

Fretts, R. C. (2001). Maternal age and fetal loss: Older women have increased risk of unexplained fetal deaths. *British Medical Journal,* 322, 430.

Friedan, B. (1963). *The Feminine mystique.* Melbourne: Dominion Press.

Friedman, S.S. (1995). Making history: reflections on feminism, narrative and desire. *Feminism beside itself.* D. Elam, & R. Weigmen. New York, Routledge.

Froman, R. D., & Owen, S. V. (1989). Infant care self efficacy. *Scholarly Inquiry for Nursing Practice,* 3, 199-211.

Gastaldo, D. (1997). Is health education good for you? In A. Petersen, & R. Bunton (Eds.), *Foucault, health and medicine* (pp. 113-133). London: Routledge.

Gastaldo, D., & Holmes, D. (1999). Foucault and nursing: A history of the present. *Nursing Inquiry,* 6, 231-240.

Geertz, C. (1963). *Old society and new states: The quest for modernity in Asia and Africa.* New York: Free Press.

Geertz, C. (1988). *Works and lives: The anthropologist as author.* Stanford, California: Stanford University Press.

Gelles, R. J., & Hargreaves, E. F. (1981). Maternal employment and violence towards children. *Journal of Family Issues,* 2(4), 509-530.

Gerard, C., Harris, K. A., & Thach, B. T. (2002). Spontaneous arousals in supine infants while swaddled and unswaddled during rapid eye movement and quiet sleep. *Pediatrics,* 110(6), 6.

Gergen, K. (2001). Self narration in social life. In M. Wetherell, S. Taylor & S. J. Yates (Eds.), *Discourse theory and practice* (pp. 247-260). Thousand Oaks: Sage.

243

Giddings, L. S., & Wood, P. J. (2002). Discourse analysis: Making connections between knowledge and power: An interview with Debbie Payne. *Nursing Praxis in New Zealand*, 18(2), 4-14.

Gjerdingen, D., McGovern, P., Bekker, M., & Willemsen, T. (2000). Women's work roles and their impact on health, well-being and career: Comparisons between the United States, Sweden and the Netherlands. *Women and Health*, 31(4), 1-20.

Glazener, C. M., Abdalla, M., Stroud, P., Naji, S., Templeton, A., & Russell, I. T. (1995). Postnatal maternal morbidity: Extent, causes, prevention and treatment. *British Journal of Obstetrics and Gynaecology*, 102, 282-287.

Glenn, E. N. (1994). Social constructions of mothering: A thematic overview. In E. N. Glenn, G. Chang & L. R. Forcey (Eds.), *Mothering ideology: Experience and agency* (pp. 1-29). London: Routledge.

Goffman, E. (1969). *The Presentation of self in everyday life*. London: Penguin.

Golden, J. (1996). *A social history of wet nursing in America: From breast to bottle*. Cambridge: Cambridge University Press.

Gornick, J. C., & Meyers, M. K. (2003). *Families that work: Policies for reconciling parenthood and employment*. New York: Russell Sage.

Gornick, V. (1996). Who says we haven't made a revolution? *New York Times Magazine*, p. 56.

Gottesman, M. M. (1992). Maternal adaptation during pregnancy among early, middle and late childbearers: Similarities and differences. *Maternal-Child Nursing Journal*, 20(2), 93-110.

Gottfried, A. E., & Gottfried, A. W. (1988). *Maternal employment and children's development: Longitudinal research*. New York: Plenum Press.

Gottlieb, L. (1978). Maternal attachment in primiparas. *Journal of Obstetric, Gynecologic, and Neonatal Nursing*, Jan/Feb, 39-44.

Graneheim, U. H., & Lundman, B., (2003). Qualitative content analysis in nursing research: concepts, procedures and measures to achieve trustworthiness. *Nurse Education Today* 24, 105-112.

Granrose, C. S., & Kaplan, E. E. (1996). *Work-family role choices for women in their 20s and 30s.* London: Praeger.

Grayzel, S. R. (1997). The mothers of our soldiers' children: Motherhood, immortality, and the war baby scandal, 1914-18. In C. Nelson & A. S. Holmes (Eds.), *Maternal instincts: Visions of motherhood and sexuality in Britain, 1875-1925* (pp. 122-140). New York: St Martin's Press.

Green, J. (2001). *Babyville*. London: Penguin.

Green, J. M. (1998). Postnatal depression or perinatal dysphoria? *Journal of Reproductive and Infant Psychology,* 16, 143-155.

Green, J. M., & Kafetsios, K. (1997). Positive experiences of early motherhood: Predictive variables from a longitudinal study. *Journal of Reproductive and Infant Psychology,* 15(2), 141-157.

Greer, G. (1970). *The female eunuch.* London: MacGibbon & Kee.

Grieve, N. (1986). The psychology of women and feminist thought: An ambivalent liaison. In N. Grieve & A. Burns (Eds.), *Australian women: New feminist perspectives* (pp. 122-141). Melbourne: Oxford University Press.

Gross, S. J., Mettelman, B. B., Dye, T. D., & Slagle, T. A. (2001). Impact of family structure and stability on academic outcome in preterm children at 10 years of age. *The Journal of Pediatrics,* 138(2), 169-175.

Grossman, F. K., Eichler, L. S., & Winickoff, S. A. (1980). *Pregnancy, birth and parenthood: Adaptation of mothers, fathers and infants*. San Francisco: Jossey-Bass.

Gubrium, F. J., & Holstein, J. A. (2000). Analyzing interpretative practice. In N. Denzin & Y. Lincoln (Eds.), *Handbook of qualitative research*, (2nd ed. pp. 487-508). London: Sage.

Hale, T. (2000). *Medications and mothers milk* (9th ed.). Amarillo: Pharmacy Medical Publishing.

Hammersley, M. (1992). *Whats wrong with ethnography?* London: Routledge.

Hanna, B., & Rolls, C. (2001). How do early parenting centres support women with an infant who has a sleep problem? *Contemporary Nurse*, 11(2/3), 153-62.

Hardin, P. K. (2001). Theory and language: Locating agency between free will and discursive marionettes. *Nursing Inquiry*, 8(1), 11-18.

Hardyment, C. (1983). *Dream babies: Three centuries of good advice on child care*. New York: Harper & Row.

Harker, L., & Thorpe, K. (1992). The last egg in the basket: Elderly primiparity, a review of the findings. *Birth*, 19(1), 23-30.

Harris, R. L., Ellicott, A. M., & Holmes, D. S. (1986). The timing of psychosocial transitions and changes in women's lives. *Journal of Personality and Social Psychology*, 51, 409-416.

Hattery, A. (2001). *Women, work and family: Balancing and weaving*. London: Sage.

Hawkins-Walsh, E., Hiscock, H., & Wake, M. (2003). A behavioral infant sleep intervention resolved infant sleep problems. *Evidence-Based Nursing*, 6(1), 10.

Hays, S. (1996). *The cultural contradictions of motherhood*. New Haven: Yale University Press.

Heck, K., Schoendorf, K. C., Ventura, S. J., & Kiely, J. L. (1997). Delayed childbearing by education level in the United States, 1969-1994. *Maternal and Child Health Journal*, 1(2), 81-88.

Hertz, R. (1997). *Reflexivity and voice.* Thousand Oaks: Sage.

Hewlett, S. A. (2002a). *Baby hunger: The new battle for motherhood.* London: Atlantic Books.

Hewlett, S. A. (2002b). *Creating a life: Professional women and the quest for children.* New York: Talk Miramax.

Hewlett, S. A. (2002c). Executive women and the myth of having it all. [Electronic version] *Harvard Business Review On Point* (product no. 9616).

Hill, P. (2000). Update on breastfeeding: Healthy people 2010 objectives. *MCN: The American Journal of Maternal / Child Nursing,* 25(5), 248-251.

Hill, P., Humenick, S. S., Argubright, T. M., & Aldag, J. C. (1997). Effects of parity and weaning practices on breastfeeding duration. *Public Health Nursing,* 14(4), 227-234.

Hiscock, H., & Wake, M. (2001). Infant sleep problems and postnatal depression: A community based study. *Pedriatrics*, 107(6), 1317-1322.

Hochschild, A. (1989). *The second shift: Working parents and the revolution at home.* New York: Viking.

Hoffman, L. W., Youngblade, L. M. (1999). *Mothers at work: Effects on children's well-being.* Cambridge: Cambridge University Press.

Hoffnung, M. (1995). Motherhood: Contemporary conflict for women. In J. Freeman (Ed.), *Women:A feminist perspective* (5th ed., pp. 162-180). California: Mayfield Publishing Company.

Hollier, L. M., Leveno, K. J., Kelly, M. A., McIntire, D. D., & Cunningham, F. G. (2000). Maternal age and malformations in singleton births. *Obstetrics and Gynecology,* 96(5), 701-706.

Holstein, J. A., & Gubrium, J. F. (2000). *The self we live by*. Oxford: Oxford University Press.

Holt, L. H. (1988). Medical perspectives on pregnancy and birth: Biological risks and technological advances. In G. Y. Michaels & W. A. Goldberg (Eds.), *Transition to parenthood: Current theory and research* (pp. 157-175). New York: Cambridge University Press.

Holsti, O. R. (1969). *Content analysis for the social sciences and humanities*. New York: Addison-Wesley.

Howard, V. (1990). *Breastfeeding handbook*. Melbourne: Lothian.

Hunt, C. E., Lesklo, S. M., Vezina, R. M., McCoy, R., Corwin, M. J., Mandell, F., et al. (2003). Infant sleep position and associated health outcomes. *Archives of Pediatrics and Adolescent Medicine*, 157(5), 496-474.

Hurst, I. (2001). Vigilant watching over: Mothers' actions to safeguard their premature babies in the newborn intensive care nursery. *The Journal of Perinatal and Neonatal Nursing*, 15(3), 39–57.

Imeson, M., & McMurray, A. (1996). Couples experiences of infertility: A phenomenological study. *Journal of Advanced Nursing*, 24(5), 1014-1022.

Jaggar, A., & Young, I. M. (2000). *A companion to feminist philosophy*. Malden, Massachussets: Blackwell.

Johnson, C. L., & Johnson, F. A. (1980). Parenthood, marriage, and careers: Situational constraints and role strain. In F. Pepitone-Rochwell (Ed.), *Dual-career couples* (pp. 143-161). London: Sage.

Kaplan, E. A. (1992). *Motherhood and representation*. London: Routledge.

Kearney, M., & Cronenwett, L. (1991). Breastfeeding and employment. *Journal of Obstetric, Gynecologic, and Neonatal Nursing*, 20(6), 471-480.

Keefe, M., Froese-Fretz, A., & Kotzer, A. M. (1998). Newborn predictors of infant irritability. *Journal of Obstetric, Gynecologic, and Neonatal Nursing,* 27(5), 513-520.

Keller, K. (1994). *Mothers and work in popular American magazines.* London: Greenwood Press.

Kerr, S. M., Jowett, S. A., & Smith, L. N. (1996). Preventing sleep problems in infants: A randomised controlled trial. *Journal of Advanced Nursing,* 24(5), 938-942.

Kitzinger, S. (1980). *Women as mothers.* New York: Vintage Books.

Kitzinger, S. (1987). *The experience of breastfeeding.* London: Penguin Books.

Klaus, M. H., & Kennell, J. H. (1976). *Maternal infant bonding.* St Louis: Mosby.

Koch, T. (1998). Story telling: Is it really research? *Journal of Advanced Nursing,* 28(6), 1182-1190.

Koch, T., & Harrington, A. (1998). Reconceptualising rigour: The case for reflexivity. *Journal of Advanced Nursing,* 28(4), 882-890.

Kong, T. S., Mahoney, D., & Plummer, K. (2002). Queering the interview. In J. F. Gubrium & J. A. Holstein (Eds.), *Handbook of interview research: Context and method* (pp. 239-258). Thousand Oaks: Sage.

Kramer, M. S., Chalmers, B., Hodnett, E. D., Sevkovskaya, Z., Dzikovich, I., Shapiro, S. et al. (2001). Promotion of breastfeeding intervention trial (PROBIT): A randomized trial in the republic of Belarus. *Journal of the American Medical Association,* 285(4), 413-420.

Kreuger, R. A. (1994). *Focus Groups / a practical guide for applied research.* Thousand Oaks: Sage.

Krippendorff, K. (1980). *Content analysis: an introduction to its methodology.* Newbury Park, Sage Publications.

Kuchner, J. F., & Porchino, J. (1988). Delayed motherhood. In B. Birns & D. F. Hay (Eds.), *The different faces of motherhood* (pp. 259-281). New York: Plenum Press.

Kullmer, U., Zygmunt, M., Munstedt, K., & Lang, U. (2000). Pregnancies in primiparous women 35 or older: Still risk pregnancies? *Geburtshilfe und Frauenheilkunde*, 60(11), 569-575.

Kurinij, N., Shiono, P. H., Ezrine, S. F., & Rhoads, G. G. (1989). Does maternal employment affect breastfeeding? *American Journal of Public Health*, 79(9), 1247-1250.

Kurstjens, S., & Wolke, D. (2001). Postnatal and non-postnatal depression in mothers: Prevalence and associations with obstetric, sociodemographic and psychosocial factors. *Zeitschrift fur Klinische Psychologie und Psychotherapie*, 30, 33-41.

Kvale, S. (1996). *Interviews: An introduction to qualitative research interviewing*. Thousand Oaks: Sage.

La Leche League (1977). *The womanly art of breastfeeding* (24th ed). Franklin Park, Illinois: Interstate Printers.

Lambden, M. P. (2001). The mediational role of working mother perceived self-efficacy. (Doctoral dissertation, University of Texas, 2001). *Digital Abstracts International, 62,* 03.

Lane, P., McKenna, H., Ryan, A. A, & Fleming, P. (2001). Focus group methodology. *Nurse Researcher*, 8(3), 45-59.

Lawrence, R. A., & Lawrence, R. M. (1999). *Breastfeeding: A guide for the medical profession* (5 ed). St Louis: Mosby.

Lawson, K., & Tulloch, M. I. (1995). Breastfeeding duration: Prenatal intentions and postnatal practices. *Journal of Advanced Nursing*, 22(5), 841-849.

Leach, P. (1975). *Babyhood: Infant development from birth to two years*. Middlesex, UK: Penguin.

Lederman, R. P. (1984). *Psychosocial adaptation in pregnancy*. Englewood Cliffs, NJ: Prentice Hall.

Lehmann, D. K., & Chism, J. (1987). Pregnancy outcome in medically complicated and uncomplicated patients aged 40 years or older. *American Journal of Obstetrics and Gynecology,* 157(3), 738-742.

Leifer, M. (1980). *Psychological effects of motherhood: A study of first pregnancy*. New York: Praeger.

Leonard, V. W. (1993). Stress and coping in the transition to parenthood of first-time mothers with career commitments: an interpretative study. (Doctoral dissertation, University of California, 1993). *Digital Abstracts International, 54*, 08.

Lerner, J. V. (1994). *Working women and their families*. Thousand Oaks: Sage.

Leucken, L. J., Suarez, E. C., Kuhn, C. M., Barefoot, J. C., Blumental, J. A., Siegler, I. C., et al. (1997). Stress in employed women: Impact of marital status and children at home on neurohormone output and home strain. *Psychosomatic Medicine*, 59(4), 352- 359.

Levinson, D. J. (1996). *The seasons of a woman's life*. New York: Knopf.

Lewis, J. (1980). *The politics of motherhood: Child and maternal welfare in England 1900-1939*. London: Croom Helm.

Lipson, J. (1991). The use of self in ethnographic research. In J. M. Morse (Ed.), *Qualitative nursing research: A contemporary dialogue* (pp. 23-43). London: Sage.

Logsdon, M. C., & Davis, D. W. (2003). Social and professional support for pregnant and parenting women. *MCN, The American Journal of Maternal / Child Nursing* , 28(6), 371-376.

Long, L. (2003). Understanding a crying baby in the first 3 months. *Community Practitioner*, 76(5), 175-81.

251

Lopata, H. (1971). *Occupation: Housewife*. New York: Oxford University Press.

Lu, M., Prentice, J., Yu, S. M., Inkelas, M., Lange, L. O., & Halfon, N. (2003). Childbirth education classes: Sociodemographic disparities in attendance and the association of attendance with breastfeeding initiation. *Maternal and Child Health Journal*, 7(2), 87-93.

Lupton, D. (1998). *The emotional self*. London: Sage.

Luthy, D. A. (1999). Maternal markers and complications of pregnancy. *The New England Journal of Medicine*, 341(27), 2085-2087.

MacArthur, C., Lewis, M., & Knox, E. G. (1991). *Health after childbirth: An investigation of long term health problems beginning after childbirth in 11071 women*. London: Her Majesty's Stationery Office.

Mahoney, C. (2000). Postnatal care scores low marks with patients. *Nursing Times*, 96(26), 20.

Mahony, R. (1995). *Kidding ourselves: Breadwinning, babies, and bargaining power*. New York: Basic Books.

Main, D. M., Main, E. K., & Moore, D. H. (2000). The relationship between maternal age and uterine dysfunction: A continuous effect throughout reproductive life. *American Journal of Obstetrics and Gynecology*, 182(6), 1312-1317.

Mansfield, N. (2000). *Subjectivity: Theories of the self from Freud to Haraway*. St Leonards, New South Wales, Australia: Allen & Unwin.

Marasco, L., Marmet, C., & Shell, E. (2000). Polycystic ovarian syndrome: A connection to insufficient milk supply? *Journal of Human Lactation*, 16 (2), 143-48.

Marshall, C., & Rossman, G. B. (1995). *Designing qualitative research* (2nd ed). Thousand Oaks: Sage.

Marshall, C., & Rossman, G. B. (1999). *Designing qualitative research* (3rd ed.). Thousand Oaks: Sage.

Marshall, Harriet. (1991). The social construction of motherhood: An analysis of childcare and parenting manuals. In A. Phoenix, A. Woollett & E. Lloyd (Eds.), *Motherhood, meanings, practices and ideologies* (pp. 66-85). London: Sage.

Marshall, Helen. (1993). *Not having children*. Melbourne: Oxford University Press.

Martin, E. (1987). *The woman in the body: A cultural analysis of reproduction*. Boston: Beacon Press.

McGovern, P., Dowd, B., Gjerdingen, D., Moscovice, I., Kochevar, L., & Lohman, W. (1997). Time off work and the postpartum health of employed women. *Medical Care,* 35(5), 507-521.

McNamara, P., Belsky, J., & Fearon, P. (2003). Infant sleep disorders and attachment: Sleep problems in infants with insecure-resistant versus insecure-avoidant attachments to mother. *Sleep and Hypnosis,* 5(1), 17-26.

McVeigh, C. (1997a). Functional status after childbirth in an Australian sample. *Journal of Obstetric, Gynecologic, and Neonatal Nursing,* 27(4), 402-409.

McVeigh, C. (1997b). Motherhood experiences from the perspectives of first-time mothers. *Clinical Nursing Research,* 6(4), 335-348.

Meisenhelder, J. B., & Meservey, P. M. (1987). Childbearing over thirty: Description and satisfaction with mothering. *Western Journal of Nursing Research*, 9, 527-541.

Mercer, R. T. (1981). A theoretical framework for studying factors that impact on the maternal role. *Nursing Research*, 30, 73-77.

Mercer, R. T. (1985). The process of maternal role attainment at one year. *Nursing Research*, 34, 198-204.

Mercer, R. T. (1986). *First-time motherhood: Experiences from teens to forties*. New York: Springer.

Miller, B. C., & Sollie, D. L. (1980). Normal stresses during the transition to parenthood. *Family Relations*, 29, 459-465.

Miller, T. (1991). *The hippies and American values*. Knoxville: University of Tennessee Press.

Mitchell, J. (1971). *Woman's estate*. New York: Vintage Books.

Monaghan, K., Braund, D., & Brodribb, W. (2001). *Compromised milk supply due to maternal factors*. (Topics in Breastfeeding, set xiii), Melbourne, Australia: Lactation Resource Centre.

Monash IVF. (2001). *The IVF program* [brochure]. Victoria, Australia: Wood. C.

Morgan, D. L. (1993). Qualitative content analysis: a guide to paths not taken. *Qualitative Health Research* 3, 112-121.

Morrison, J., Najman, J. M., Williams, G. M., Keeping, J. D., & Anderson, H. R. (1989). Socio-economic status and pregnancy outcome: An Australian study. *British Journal of Obstetrics and Gynaecology, 96*, 298-307.

Morse, J. (1991). Qualitative nursing research, a free for all. In J. M. Morse (Ed.), *Qualitative nursing research: A contemporary dialogue* (pp. 126-145). London: Sage.

Muggli, E., & Halliday, J. (2003). *Report on prenatal diagnostic testing in Victoria 2002*. Melbourne, Australia: Murdoch Children's Research Institute.

Mulhall, A., LeMay, A., & Alexander, C. (1999). Bridging the research-practice gap: A reflective account of research work. Nt Research, 4(2), 119-131.

Muller, M. (1996). Prenatal and postnatal attachment: A modest correlation. *Journal of Obstetric, Gynecologic, and Neonatal Nursing* 25(2): 161-166.

Myles, M. F. (1985). *Textbook for midwives with modern concepts of obstetric and neonatal care.* Edinburgh: Churchill Livingstone.

Najman, J., Lanyon, A., Andersen, M., Williams, G., Bor, W., & O'Callaghan, M. (1998). Socioeconomic status and maternal cigarette smoking before, during and after a pregnancy. *Australian and New Zealand Journal of Public Health, 22*(1), 60-66.

National Centre for Epidemiology and Population Health (1998). *The Economic value of breastfeeding in Australia* (NCEPH working paper number 40). Canberra: Smith, J. P., Ingham, L. H., & Dunstone, M. D.

Navaie-Waliser, M., Martin, S. L., Tessaro, I., Campbell, M. K., & Cross, A. W. (2000). Social support and psychological functioning among high risk mothers: The impact of the baby love maternal outreach worker program. *Public Health Nursing, 17*(4), 280-291.

Neifert, M. R., Seacat, J. M., & Jobe, W. E. (1985). Lactation failure due to insufficient glandular development of the breast. *Pediatrics, 76* (5), 823- 828.

Nelson, A. M. (2003a). Older first-time mothering: Readiness and planned intensity. (Doctoral dissertation, University of Connecticut, 2003). *Digital Abstracts International, 64,* 02.

Nelson, A. M. (2003b). Transition to motherhood. *Journal of Obstetric, Gynecologic, and Neonatal Nursing, 32*(4), 465-477.

Neurgarten, B., & Datan, N. (1973). Sociological perspectives on the life cycle. In P. B. Baltes & K.W. Schaie (Eds.), *Life span development psychology: Personality and socialization* (pp. 53-69). New York: Academic press.

New, C. (1998). Realism, deconstruction and the feminist standpoint. *Journal for the Theory of Social Behavior, 28*(4), 349-372.

Nicholson, P. (1998). *Post-natal depression: Psychology, science and the transition to motherhood.* London: Routledge.

Nolan, M. (1997). Pre-natal education: Failure to educate for parenthood. *British Journal of Midwifery,* 5(1), 21-26.

Oakley, A. (1974). *Housewife.* London: A. Lane.

Oakley, A. (1979). *Becoming a mother.* Oxford: Martin Robertson.

Oakley, A. (1981). Interviewing women: A contradiction in terms. In H. Roberts (Ed.), *Doing feminist research* (pp. 30-61). London: Routledge & Kegan Paul.

Oakley, A. (1984). *The captured womb: A history of the medical care of pregnant women.* Oxford: Blackwell.

Oakley, A. (1986). *From here to maternity: Becoming a mother.* Harmondsworth, UK: Penguin.

Oakley, A. (1992). *Social support and motherhood.* Oxford: Blackwell.

Okely, J. (1992). Anthropology and autobiography: Participatory experience and embodied knowledge. In J. Okely & H. Galloway (Eds.), *Anthropology and autobiography* (pp. 1-28). London: Routledge.

Olson, A. L., & DiBrigida, L. A. (1994). Depressive symptoms and work role satisfaction in mothers of toddlers. *Pediatrics,* 94(3), 363- 367.

Orona, C. J. (1990). Temporality and identity loss due to Altzeimer's disease. *Social Science and Medicine,* 30(11), 1247-1256.

Ozer, E. M. (1995). The impact of childcare responsibility and self-efficacy on the psychological health of professional working mothers. *Psychology of Women Quarterly,* 19, 315-335.

Patton, M. Q. (1990). *Qualitative evaluation and research methods* (2nd ed.) Newbury Park: Sage.

Patton, M. Q. (2002). *Qualitative research & evaluation methods*. Thousand Oaks, Sage Publications.

Payne, D. (2002). *The elderly primigravida: Contest and complexity*. Unpublished Doctoral thesis in Nursing. Massey University, Palmerston North, New Zealand.

Peipert, J., & Bracken, M. (1993). Maternal age: An independent risk factor for caesarean delivery. *Obstertrics and Gynecology*, 81, 200-205.

Peters, J. K. (1998). *When mothers work: Loving our children without sacrificing ourselves*. Adelaide, Australia: Hodder.

Pleck, J. H. (1985). *Working wives / working husbands*. Beverley Hills: Sage.

Polit, D. F., & Hungler, B. P. (1993). *Essentials of nursing research*. Philadelphia: Lippincott.

Pollock, J. I. (1996). Mature maternity: Long term associations in first children born to older mothers in 1970 in the UK. *Journal of Epidemiology and Community Health*, 50(4), 429- 435.

Pollock, L. A. (1983). *Forgotten children: Parent-child relations from 1500 to 1900*. Cambridge: Cambridge University press.

Porter, C. L., & Hsu, H. C. (2003). First-time mothers' perceptions of efficacy during the transition to motherhood: Links to infant temperament. *Journal of Family Psychology*, 17(1), 54-64.

Pridham, K. F., & Chang, A. S. (1992). Transition to being the mother of a new infant in the first 3 months: Maternal problem solving and self appraisals. *Journal of Advanced Nursing*, 17, 204-216.

Pridham, K. F., Lytton, D., Chang, A. S., & Rutledge, D. (1991). Early postpartum transition: Progress in maternal identity and role attainment. *Research in Nursing and Health* 14: 21-31.

257

Prysak, M., Lorenz, R. P., & Kisly, A. (1995). Pregnancy outcome in nulliparous women 35 years and older. *Obstetrics and Gynecology*, 85(1), 65-70.

Pugh, L. C., & Milligan, R. M. (1993). A framework for the study of childbearing fatigue. *Advances in Nursing Science*, 15, 60-70.

Ragozin, A. S., Basham, K. A., Crnic, M. T., & Robinson, N. M. (1982). Effects of maternal age on parenting role. *Developmental Psychology*, 18(4), 627-634.

Rankin, E. A. (1993). Stresses and rewards experienced by employed mothers. *Health Care for Women International*, 14(6), 527-537.

Raphael-Leff, J. (1991). *Psychological processes of child-bearing*. London: Chapman & Hall.

Raum, E., Arabin, B., Schlaud, M., Walter, U., & Schwartz, F.W. (2001). The impact of maternal education on intrauterine growth: A comparison of former West and East Germany. *International Journal of Epidemiology*, 30, 81-87.

Razack, S. (1993). Story-telling for social change. *Gender and Education* 5(1), 55-70.

Reece, S. M. (1995). Stress and maternal adaptation in first-time mothers more than 35 years old. *Applied Nursing Research*, 8(2), 61-66.

Reinharz, S. (1992). *Feminist research methods in social research*. Oxford: Oxford University Press.

Rice, P. L., & Ezzy, D. (1999). *Qualitative research methods: A health focus*. Melbourne: Oxford University Press.

Rich, A. (1977). *Of Woman Born*. London, Virago.

Richman, A. L., Miller, P. M., & LeVine, R. A. (1992). Cultural and educational variations in maternal responsiveness. *Developmental Psychology, 28*(4), 614-621.

Righetti-Veltema, M., Conne-Perreard, E., Bousquet, A., & Manzano, J. (1998). Risk factors and predictive signs of postpartum depression. *Journal of Affective Disorders,* 49, 167-180.

Riley, D. (1988). *Am I that name? feminism and the category of 'women' in history.* London, Macmillan.

Roberts, C. L., Algert, C. S. & March, L. M. (1994). Delayed childbearing, are there any risks? *Medical Journal of Australia,* 160, 539-44.

Robson, C. (2002). *Real world research: a resource for social scientists and practitioner-researchers.* Oxford, UK: Blackwell.

Rogan, F., Schmied, V., Barclay, L., Everitt, L., & Wyllie, A. (1997). Becoming a mother: Developing a new theory of early motherhood. *Journal of Advanced Nursing,* 25(5), 877-885.

Rojjanasrirat, W. (2000). The effects of nursing intervention on breastfeeding duration among primiparous mothers planning to return to work. (Doctoral dissertation, University of Kansas, 2000). *Digital Abstracts International, 61,* 12.

Rosenwald, G. C., & Ochberg, R.L. (1992). *Storied lives: The cultural politics of self understanding.* New Haven: Yale University Press.

Rossi, A.S. (1968). Transition to parenthood. *Journal of Marriage and the family,* 30, 26- 39.

Rossi, A. S. (1980). Life span theory and women's lives. *Signs: Journal of Women in Culture and Society,* 6, 4-32.

Rothman, B. K. (1994). *The tentative pregnancy: amniocentesis and the sexual politics of motherhood.* London: Pandora.

259

Rowe, J. (2003). A room of their own: The social landscape of infant sleep. *Nursing Inquiry*, 10(3), 184-192.

Roxburgh, S. (1997). The effect of children on the mental health of women in the paid work force. *Journal of Family Issues*, 18(3), 270-289.

Rubenstein, C. (1998). *The sacrificial mother: loving your children without losing yourself.* Rydalmere, NSW, Hodder.

Rubin, R. (1967a). Attainment of the maternal role, part 1, processes. *Nursing Research*, 16, 237- 245.

Rubin, R. (1967b). Attainment of the maternal role, part 2. Models and referrants. Nursing Research, 16, 342-346.

Rubin, R. (1984). *Maternal identity and the maternal experience.* New York: Springer

Sandelowski, M. (1986). Rigor or rigor mortis: The problem of rigor in qualitative research. *Advances in Nursing Science*, 8(3), 27-37.

Sandelowski, M. (1991). Telling stories: Narrative approaches in qualitative research. *Image: Journal of Nursing Scholarship*, 23, 161-166.

Sandelowski, M. (1993). Rigor or rigor mortis: The problem of rigor in qualitative research revisited. *Advances in Nursing Science*, 16(2), 1-8.

Sandelowski, M. (1994). We are the stories we tell: Narrative knowing in nursing practice. *Journal of Holistic Nursing*, 12(1), 23-33.

Sandelowski, M. (1995a). A theory of the transition to parenthood of infertile couples. *Research in Nursing and Health*, 18, 123-132.

Sandelowski, M. (1995b). Focus on qualitative methods: Sample size in qualitative research. *Research in Nursing and Health*, 18, 179-183.

Scher, A., & Dror, E. (2003). Attachment, caregiving and sleep: The tie that keeps infants and mothers awake. *Sleep and Hypnosis,* 5(1), 27-37.

Schmied, V., & Lupton, D. (2001). The externality of the inside: Body images of pregnancy. *Nursing Inquiry*, 8(1), 32-40.

Scott, D. (1997). The researcher's personal responses as a source of insight in the research process. *Nursing Inquiry*, 4, 130-134.

Scott, D., Brady, S., & Glynn, P. (2001). New mothers groups as a social network intervention: Consumer and maternal and child health perspectives. *Journal of Advanced Nursing,* 18(4), 23-29.

Scott, J. W. (1992). Experience. *Feminists theorize the political.* J. Butler, & J. Scott, New York, Routledge: 22-40.

Scott, J. W. (1996). *Feminism and history.* New York, Oxford University Press.

Secret, M. C. (1994). The influence of work status on the psychological and social well-being of married mothers. (Doctoral dissertation, Virginia Commonwealth University, 1994). *Digital Abstracts International, 55,* 07.

Sethi, S. (1995). The dialectic in becoming a mother: Experiencing a post partum phenomenon. *Scandinavian Journal of Caring science,* 9, 235-244.

Sheridan, S., Baird, B., Borrett, K., & Ryan, L. (2002). *Who was that woman: The Australian Women's Weekly in the postwar years.* Sydney: University of New South Wales Press.

Shorter, E. (1976). *The making of the modern family*. London: Collins.

Sibai, B. M., Ewell, M., Levine, R. J., Klebanoff, M. A., Esterlitz, J., Catalano, P. M., et al. (1997). Risk factors associated with pre-eclampsia in healthy nulliparous women. *American Journal of Obstetrics and Gynecology*, 177, 1003-1010.

Singh, D., Newburn, M., Smith, N., & Wiggins, M. (2002). The information needs of first-time pregnant mothers. *British Journal of Midwifery*, 10(1), 54-58.

Smart, C. (1996). Deconstructing motherhood. In E. Bortolaia Silva (Ed.), *Good Enough Mothering* (pp. 37-58). London: Routledge.

Smit, Y., Scherjon, S. A., & Treffers, P. E. (1997). Elderly nulliparae in midwifery care in Amsterdam. *Midwifery*, 13, 73-77.

Smith, J. A. (1999). Identity development during the transition to motherhood: An interpretative phenomenological analysis. *Journal of Reproductive and Infant Psychology*, 17(3), 281-299.

Smith-Pierce, S. (1994). Juggling: A heuristic study of first-time midlife mothers (Doctoral dissertation, Union Institute, 1994). *Dissertations Abstracts International, 55*, 04B.

Speciale, H. J., & Carpenter, D. R. (2003). *Qualitative research in nursing: Advancing the humanistic imperative*. Philadelphia: Lippincott.

Spellacy, W. N., Miller, S. J., & Winegar, A. (1986). Pregnancy after 40 years of age. *Obstetrics and Gynecology*, 68, 452-454.

St James-Roberts, I., Conroy, S., & Wishler, K. (1996). Bases for maternal perceptions of infant crying and colic behaviour. *Archives of Disease in Childhood*, 75(5), 375-384.

St. Pierre, E., & Pillow, W. (2000). *Working the ruins: feminist poststructural theory and methods in education*. New York: Routledge.

Stacey (1991). Can there be a feminist ethnography? In S. B. Gluck, & D. Patai, (Eds) *Women's words: the feminist practice of oral history* (pp. 111-119). New York: Routledge.

Stark, M. A. (1997). Psychosocial adjustment during pregnancy: The experience of mature gravidas. *Journal of Obstetric, Gynecologic, and Neonatal Nursing,* 26(2), 206-211.

Stein, Z., & Susser, M. (2000). The risks of having children in later life: Social advantage may make up for biological disadvantage. *British Medical Journal,* 320(7251), 1681-1682.

Steinberg, S. I., & Bellevance, F. (1999). Characteristics and treatment of women with pre-natal and postpartum depression. *International Journal of Psychiatry in Medicine,* 20, 209-233.

Stoppard, M. (1983). *Dr Miriam Stoppard's baby care book.* London: Dorling Kindersley.

Stowe, Z. N., & Nemeroff, C. B. (1995). Women at risk for postpartum-onset major depression. *American Journal of Obstetrics and Gynecology,* 173, 639-645.

Summerfield, P. (1998). *Reconstructing women's wartime lives.* Manchester: Manchester University Press.

Sykes, G. (1999). The role of sleep clinics in helping children get a good night's sleep. *Community Nurse,* 5(9), 13-14.

Tan, K. T., & Tan, K. H. (1994). Pregnancy and delivery in primigravidae aged 35 and older. *Singapore Medical Journal,* 35, 495-501.

Tarkka, M. T. (2003). Predictors of maternal competence by first-time mothers when the child is 8 months old. *Journal of Advanced Nursing,* 41(3), 233–240.

Tarkka, M. T., & Paunonen, M. (1996). Social support and its impact on mothers' experiences of childbirth. *Journal of Advanced Nursing,* 23(1), 70-75.

263

Tarkka, M. T., Paunonen, M., & Laippala, P. (1999). Social support provided by public health nurses and the coping of first-time mothers with child care. *Public Health Nursing,* 16(2), 114-119.

Teutsch, D. (2002, July 07). Caesarean or I'll sue! Melbourne, Australia: *Sun Herald,* p. 5.

Thurer, S. L. (1994). *The myths of motherhood.* New York, Houghton Mifflin.

Tulman, L. J. (1981). Theories of maternal attachment. *Advances in Nursing Science,* (July), 7-14.

Turner, J. C. (1987). *Rediscovering the social group: A self categorization theory.* Oxford: Basil Blackwell.

Twiss, J. J. G. (1989). The effect of first-time childbearing on women 35 years or older as compared to younger women: The transition difficulty, maternal adaptations and role satisfactions. (Doctoral dissertation, University of Nebraska, 1989). *Digital Abstracts International, 51,* 03.

U.K. National Statistics (2001). *Social Trends* (no 31). London: Her Majesty's Stationery Office: Church, J., Jackson, J., Jackson,V., Kerskaw, A., Lillistone, C., Manners, A. M. et al.

U.S. Center for Disease Control and Prevention. (2001a). *Births: Final data for 1999,* (National Vital Statistics Report volume 49, No. 1. (PHS) 2001-1120). Atlanta, GA: Ventura, S. J., Martin, J.A. & Curtin, S.C.

U.S. Center for Disease Control and Prevention. (2001b). *Trends in pregnancy rates for the United States, 1976-97, An update* (National Vital Statistics Report. Vol. 49, No. 4. 10 pp. (PHS) 2001-1120). Hyatsville, Maryland: Ventura, S. J., Mosher, W. D., Curtin, S. C., Abma, J. C., & Henshaw, S.

van der Wal, M. F., van den Boom, D. C., Pauw-Plomp, H., & de Jonge, G. A. (1998). Mothers' reports of infant crying and soothing in a multicultural population. *Archives of Disease in Childhood,* 79(4), 312-317.

Ventura, S. J. (1989). First births to older mothers. *American Journal of Public Health,* 79, 1675.

Viau, P. A., Padula, C., & Eddy, B. (2002). An exploration of the health concerns and health promotion behaviours in pregnant women over age 35. *The American Journal of Maternal / Child Nursing,* 27(6), 328-334.

Visness, C. M., & Kennedy, K. I. (1997). Maternal employment and breastfeeding: Findings from the 1988 National Maternal and Infant Health Survey. *American Public Health Association,* 87(6), 945-950.

Wagner, V. (1995). In the name of feminism. In D. Elam, & R. Weigmen (Eds). *Feminism beside itself* (pp.119-131). New York: Routledge.

Wall, S. N., Khoshnood, B., Singh, J. K., Hsieh, H. & Lee, K. (1998). Multilevel analysis of the effects of low-income residence on the risk of lbw associated with   advanced maternal age in African Americans and Whites (supplement 2). *Paediatric Research,* 43(4), 233.

Walzer, J. F. (1976). A period of ambivalence: Eighteenth century American childhood. In L. deMause (Ed.), *The history of childhood* (pp. 351-382). London: Souvenir Press.

Walzer, S. (1998). *Thinking about the baby: Gender and transitions into parenthood.* Philadelphia: Temple University Press.

Warner, R., Appleby, L., Whitton, A., & Faragher, B. (1996). Demographic and obstetric risk factors for postnatal psychiatric morbidity. *British Journal of Psychiatry,* 168, 607-611.

Wasserfall, R. R. (1997). Reflexivity, feminism and difference. In R. Hertz (Ed.), *Reflexivity and voice* (pp. 150-168). Thousand Oaks: Sage.

Weingarten, K. (1994). *The mother's voice: Strengthening intimacy in families.* New York: Harcourt Brace.

Weiss, G. (1999). *Body images: embodiment as intercorporeality.* New York: Routledge.

West, P. (1990). The status and validity of accounts obtained at interview: A contrast between two studies of families with a disabled child. *Social Science and Medicine,* 30(11), 1229-1239.

White, H. (1981). The value of narrativity in the representation of reality. In W. J. T. Mitchell (Ed.), *On narrative* (pp. 1-24). Chicago: Chicago University Press.

Why I don't like working with mothers. (2001, Dec). *SHE,* 43-44.

Wildschut, H. I. J. (1999). Sociodemographic factors: Age, parity, social class and ethnicity. In D. K. James, P. J. Steer, C. P. Weiner & B. Gonik (Eds.), *High risk pregnancy* (2nd ed., pp. 39-52). London: W.B. Saunders.

Wilk, C. A. (1986). *Career women and childbearing.* New York: Van Nostrand Reinhold.

Willinger, M., Ko, C., Hoffman, H. J., Kessler, R. C., & Corwin, M. C. (2003). Trends in bed sharing in the United States, 1993-2000: The national infant sleep position study. *Archives of Pediatrics and Adolescent Medicine,* 157(1), 49-9.

Windridge, K. C., & Berryman, J.C. (1996). Maternal adjustment and maternal attitudes during pregnancy and early motherhood in women of 35 and older. *Journal of Reproductive and Infant Psychology,* 14, 45-55.

Windridge, K. C., & Berryman, J. C. (1999). Women's experience of giving birth after 35. *Birth,* 26(1), 16-23.

Wolke, D., Sohne, B., Reigel, K., Ohrt, B., & Osterlund, K. (1998). An epidemiological longitudinal study of sleeping problems and feeding experience of preterm and term children in southern Finland: Comparison with a southern German population sample. *The Journal of Pediatrics,* 133(2), 224-231.

World Health Organisation (1991). *Infant feeding; the physiological basis* (Bulletin 67, supplement). Geneva.

World Health Organisation (2002). *Nutrient adequacy of exclusive breastfeeding for the term infant during the first six months of life*. Geneva: Butte, N. F., Lopez-Alarcon, M. G., & Cutberto, G.

Wrightsman, L. S. (1988). *Personality development in adults*. London: Sage.

Yankelovich, D. (1974). *The new morality: A profile of American youth in the 70's*. New York: McGraw-Hill.

Zybert, P., Stein, Z., & Belmont, L. (1978). Maternal age and children's ability. *Percept Motor Skills, 47*, 815-818.

Appendix A

Themes for interview

Question/themes for interviews

INTERVIEW 1 [prenatal interview]

- Demographic information: Age, educational status, work, duration of current relationship

- Why/how did you decide to have a baby now, at this point in your life?

- How have you prepared for the birth of your baby?

- How do you feel about the forthcoming birth?

- Do you feel prepared for the birth?

INTERVIEW 2

- How was the birth?

- How did your expectations of birth match the reality of labour and delivery?

- Do you feel you were well prepared for the birth?

- What/ if anything would have made a difference to your experience of birth?

INTERVIEW 3

- How have you adjusted to your parenting role?

- What lifestyle changes, if any, have you made since the arrival of your baby?

- What information, if any, would have made the adjustment easier?

- How well did your expectations match the reality of your role as a new mother?

Appendix B

Overview of study themes / feedback from participants

Overview of study themes / feedback from participants

Before and during pregnancy

- Deciding to have a baby
- Becoming well informed/ internet/ books/ medical information
- Getting really healthy
- Making choices about type of hospital/ care
- Choosing a doctor
- Making plans
- Setting up work and home
- Keeping the pregnancy quiet
- Not wanting to be seen in a different light

Comments:

Overview of study themes / feedback from participants

First few weeks
It's a nightmare in the beginning

Overwhelming/ exhausting:

- Never any time/ constant/draining
- Sheer volume of work/ domestics
- Losing independence
- Isolated at home
- Out of my control
- Feeling anxious
- Very worried about the baby
- Afraid to sleep or shower and leave the baby unattended

Comments:

Overview of study themes / feedback from participants

4-12 weeks
It's a struggle

> - My whole life is changing/
> - Not my life any more
> - Feeling really unsure
> - Not wanting to change too much
> - Wanting to hang on to something of me
> - Realizing the task is a long standing one/
> - Wondering did I make the right decision
> - Trying to find my own way

Comments:

Overview of study themes / feedback from participants

4-6 months
Giving in/ letting go

Giving in because things work better if the baby has naps at home
Letting go of things- just too much hassle to continue with previous life
Realising people 'just don't do it' [take babies out all the time]

Things getting better:
Baby more interactive
Breakthroughs/ getting to know the baby
Recognising the cues

Realising:
- that the baby is not so fragile
- that it's OK to have negative feelings
- that you can't 'do it all'
- realising that there is no one right way

Finding my own way

Comments:

Overview of study themes / feedback from participants

Feeling like a mother- 6-8 months

- Liking it more/recommend it highly
- Changing priorities/ this is what is really important
- Missing the baby when I'm away/ different than just worrying
- The baby has become my job
- Finding the balance, between work and family life
- Thinking about what it means to be an older mother
- Worrying about my future health and lifespan

Comments:

Appendix C

Themes for focus group discussion

Focus group data and findings

Focus Groups

Although the primary focus of this work has been the maternal experiences of primiparae aged greater than 35 years, three focus groups of midwives and M&CHNs were also conducted. The information gathered at focus groups, it was anticipated, would assist in framing the research question and provide useful background for the study. As my interest in this field had emerged from my clinical role, I also needed to test my views and assumptions against those of my colleagues, in a bid to understand their experiences of this cohort. Did they see primiparae over 35 as a distinct cohort? What did they understand to be the issues and challenges facing this group of mothers? The clinical care requirements for this group of women was another subject of interest as it was my understanding that primiparae aged greater than 35 had needs that differed from other groups of mothers.

Of the three focus groups conducted, two were composed of hospital-based midwives and a single mothercraft nurse employed at the hospital where the women gave birth. The third focus group consisted of community-based maternal and child health nurses local to the hospital. Themes for discussion included:

How do we as midwives and maternal and child health nurses view older first-time mothers?

- Are they a distinct group?
- If so, how are they different?
- Do they have specific needs?
- If so, what are those specific needs?
- Do older primiparae require care that differs from other mother?
- If so how does it differ?

Rationale: why focus groups?

In general, focus groups are considered to be useful when participants share certain characteristics relevant to a particular study (Marshall & Rossman, 1995; Speciale & Carpenter, 2003) as in this case, when all participants were involved in the care of primiparae over 35 years. Another strength of this format is its social orientation, which tends to promote group interaction (Lane, McKenna, Ryan & Fleming, 2001). Furthermore, this format allowed the interviewer to probe and thus elicit more in-depth information (Kreuger, 1994). Finally, in line with the post-structural understanding that an individual's attitudes do not form in isolation, but through interaction with others, focus group interaction was considered a useful and congruent means here, to gain additional insight into the phenomenon of mothering when aged over 35.

Recruitment and conduct

Recruitment of focus group participants occurred over a two-week period and information posters were displayed at the hospital maternity unit and at several adjacent Maternal and Child Health Centres [M&CHCs], inviting interest and outlining time commitments of focus group participation. The researcher's telephone number was included for expression of interest and clarification of detail. Theme lists were provided prior to the focus group in a bid to reduce concerns and to encourage reflection on the themes for discussion. To facilitate the midwives' convenience, focus groups were conducted on site in the hospital. The M&CHN focus group was conducted in a local M&CHC. Six participants attended each group. All sessions were audiotaped.

Findings

Findings are divided into the following sub-sections:

- Nursing attitudes to later timing
- Care requirements /Particular concerns
- Older primiparae as a challenging group
- Dealing with the dilemmas of older primiparae

- Possible solutions

Nursing (Midwifery and M&CHN) attitudes to later timing

Data from the midwifery and to a lesser extent M&CHN focus groups, supported social attitudes of later parenting, as commonly articulated in discourses. The following quotes represent the midwives' reactions to hearing that a 45-year-old primipara was to be admitted that day:

Oh MY God, you're too old to be having a baby…

45 it's too … too old! They're too over the top sometimes. First of all, what are you doing having a baby at this age! Is it just … you know like …to have a baby to complete the circle … like you've had your career … you're married … you've got your house, then the baby comes … closed book!

Well, I wouldn't think of having a baby at 45, put it that way! It's too old!

This is the last thing on the agenda!

They're mad! … Who'd want to do it? Suppose you're nearly at change of life, they think they better have it now! Mid life crisis! The old clock has suddenly started ticking!

Babies for the older group, are an accessory as well, you hear them, it sounds terrible but, they've got the Emmalunga pram and the new baby, they've got the beautiful house with the two BMWs, what we need is the pram and the baby!

In general, the comments reflect social impressions of career women selfishly pursuing career and financial considerations before finally having a baby, as the 'last thing on the agenda'. The hospital midwives, although kind and empathetic to the women publicly, were often privately disparaging of the women's 'selfish' choices around career and family. Value judgments of 'being too old', 'mad' or suffering a 'mid-life crisis' are made, though there is a general tendency by the midwives to try and 'give them what they needed', in terms of help and support postpartum. In general, however, the midwives often saw the mothers as time-consuming and demanding, compared to other patients. The following comments indicate the midwives' views:

Oh you think, this'll be a lot of work!

I think you have to give them more time, as midwives ...

She's going to end up with PND! [Postnatal depression]

They are at more of a loss they expect, I feel they (older mothers) actually expect more of us they want things to be perfect, a lot more than other women want them to be ...

Constantly striving for perfection. I must express at 11 minutes past five ... and now its 12 minutes past, where is the pump?

They're focused on every book they can read!

The gut feeling is gone ... disconnected, the natural feeling is gone!

In contrast, M&CHNs were more positive about the older primiparae, as evidenced by their commentary, though they too recognised maternal characteristics such as vulnerability, striving for perfection and focusing on extensive literature. The M&CHNs also tended to recognise the strengths of this group, but nonetheless associated them with high levels of postnatal depression and maladjustment:

Anxious higher expectations! Unrealistic expectations!

They've done a lot of reading ...

Very well-educated usually, career focused ...

I just wonder whether they've already got the subconscious notion about themselves as well? Performance anxiety?

I'm always thinking about older women and associating them with PND. A lot of them have PND! Or those sorts of conditions!

Care requirements/ Particular concerns

There was a general suggestion by both midwives and M&CHNs of poorer performance with breastfeeding, poorer tolerance of sleep disturbance, higher levels of anxiety and a pre-occupation with infant sleeping patterns, which is quite closely aligned to findings of the current study. The following

quotes are representative:

Breastfeeding:

> *I expect them to be baaaaad at breastfeeding! It doesn't come across as real natural for them! Whether they have missed the boat by having the baby, naturally!! Physically? Like physically their body's not performing...*
>
> [Midwife]

> *When I hear that someone is 43 just had her first baby, I think breastfeeding, that's my first thought ... They just don't lactate as well!*
>
> [M&CHN]

> *And they sort of ... and they can't get comfy and their baby's not right and they look awkward and they never look as if they're doing it as naturally as someone in their twenties or early thirties would do it ... you seldom see them sling on the baby, that's what I've noticed...*   [M&CHN]

Sleeping:

> *Sleeping consumes them, 'how long'... 'Does your baby sleep through? ... And they just ... They need the baby to sleep, it's just a real thing, isn't it?*
>
> [M&CHN]

> *So they measure how good a mother they are by how much it sleeps, by how settled their baby is...*   [M&CHN]

Anxiety

> *I feel that these mothers have an anxiety problem, not so much a problem but a situation that arises and it peaks at about 8 weeks and then it seems to drop by about 4 months ...*
> [M&CHN]

> *The more anxious they are ... they are more needy!*   [Midwife]

Although in general, the older primiparae were seen as anxious and needy, some exceptions are

expressed and this trend is more common among the M&CHNs. Della (M&CHN) found that older

281

mothers were often resourceful and were possessed of other skills and Cathy (M&CHN) felt that older

mothers were sometimes 'more together in themselves' in terms of selfhood.

They often have lots of skills they can draw on!
Della [M&CHN]

They're sometimes a bit more together in themselves, based on who they are because we all sort of develop our identity as we grow older, don't we?
Cathy [M&CHN]

Della also found that primiparae over 35 presented varying degrees of capability and discussed seeing a

whole range of differences among these women:

I've found they're anxious [but] I certainly get some elderly primips that have been very capable Not super-anxious, I mean, they had their concerns but one of them was 41 or 42 when she had her first baby, coz I remember thinking 'oh, I wonder how she will go...Oh, she had her little hiccups, but she was no worse than anybody else... [M&CHN]

Older primiparae as a challenging group

Both groups of health professionals found the women's depth of knowledge challenging and worried

about the best way to offer advice. Some paced their advice to what the mother already knew and

strove to avoid offering 'conflicting advice'. Others worried about the possibility of 'missing

something' as they trod carefully around the mothers' sensibilities:

I approach them with trepidation; I listen for cues about what she is wanting to do and try to match my approach to what she is saying ...
[Midwife]

I find it actually quite daunting [looking after them] A bit confronting! I find them challenging too! And if you say something she doesn't quite agree with you know quite quickly that she's not very happy about it. I've thought a lot about the way I approach it with her ... I have developed a lot more skills with asking her 'what would you like to do? What have you been doing?
[M&CHN]

The only thing I felt a bit ... was I missing things because I didn't want to step on her toes too much ...   [M&CHN]

They seem to go to many places to try and find the 'right' solution, so they may not have only come here to me, but then you might find 'I've rung them and they told me this and I've asked this person and they've told me this so by the time they get to you, you think "what am I going to tell you that's going to help here?"
[M&CHN]

In this study, the midwives tended to be privately dismissive of the older mothers' concerns, particularly minor worries and attention to detail such as 'how long should I burp my baby for? They did, however, care for the women kindly. In contrast, the M&CHNs seemed to go to considerably more effort to elicit the source of the woman's knowledge and work out what might help. The midwives' attitudes can perhaps be explained by their busy workloads and also by the fact that the facility in which they worked also cared for seriously ill pregnant women, some of whom had life-threatening conditions. In this tertiary level hospital where most of the older mothers choose to, or were advised to, give birth, the minor concerns and time-consuming questions of the older primiparae were given little priority by the midwives when compared to other 'real' concerns. Additionally, the midwives first came upon the mothers 'at their worst', in the fatigue-filled and anxiety-laden days of early motherhood. There was limited time to establish a rapport, with most of the women attending a private obstetrician for their pregnancy care. In contrast, the M&CHNs came in contact with the mothers several days later and in the comfort and familiarity of the woman's own home. This differing environment perhaps accounts for disparities noted between the midwives and M&CHNs' attitudes. Additionally, the M&CHNs had the added benefit of seeing the mothers improve and accommodate the transition to motherhood over a longer period of time, whereas the midwives tended to care for women only in the immediate peri-natal period.

As I wrote this passage, I felt an extraordinary need to defend the remarks of my midwifery colleagues, as not truly representative of the service they provide. I am aware of the thousand small kindnesses they individually and collectively perform for these mothers, many of which are well beyond the call of duty. One colleague, a lactation consultant, often visits these mothers, out of hours, without monetary gain, to assist with particular feeding difficulties. All of the midwives invite anxious mothers to call the unit for advice and regularly arrange for a mother to return for breastfeeding advice or to weigh her baby if worried. For particular concerns, 'casual' domiciliary visits are made to 'check how she's going'. There is a clearly understood philosophy of wanting the mothers to 'do well'. Upon further reflection, I realise that despite having a well-defined interest in the needs of the older primiparae, I too identify with the midwives' comments and have often stifled a sigh of reluctance when asked to care for an older mother, prior exposure to whom has made me realise that she will consume much of my shift, leaving me little time to attend to my four other patients.

Dealing with the dilemmas of older primiparae

You just have to handle them differently!   Cathy [M&CHN]

The dilemmas and concerns of the older primiparae received different attention by both midwives and M&CHNs involved in their care, when compared to younger mothers or women having a second or subsequent child. The midwives commonly described attending to their other patients first, lest they get 'tied up' with the time-consuming issues of the older primipara, such as breastfeeding or routine care of the infant. Most midwives went to efforts to establish a rapport with the woman and to systematically deal with her concerns. Ancillary services such as lactation consultants, paediatric visits and physiotherapy referrals were also called upon with greater frequency for this group. Despite ever-earlier hospital discharge, the midwives often negotiated for an extra day in hospital for the older primiparae. Maternal and child health nurses also frequently described allocating extra time to older primiparae, usually allowing an hour for the mother's first visit instead of the more usual half hour. Often they would organise to see the women more frequently, at least initially. Cathy and Della [M&CHNs] explain:

284

And I think that I actually do see women more often who I think they're more vulnerable ... I do I probably see them weekly for quite a while!

If she was older, certainly I would ... like an alarm bell ... it'll be a long home visit, it'll take the whole hour!

Some went to considerable effort establishing their credentials with the mothers, prior to proceeding with the visit. Here, Betty (M&CHN) describes speaking of conferences she had attended and offering expert opinion to support her suggestions of infant care:

We're continually going on seminars and I think they respond really well to you saying 'well, I attended this seminar with this particular doctor, this gastro-enterologist and his view on that was' ... they seem to really quite like that!

Cathy [M&CHN] draws on her experiences at an established mother and baby unit:

Coz when they're moving into solids and that kind of stuff, I can talk about some experiences I had at the 'O'Connell Centre' and infant feeding...

Possible solutions

There was a consistent finding of too few maternal skills at the time of discharge from hospital and most M&CHNs felt that the mothers would benefit from an additional day or two in hospital, to equip them with parenting skills and to assist with establishing lactation. There was a clearly articulated understanding that not all mothers would require this level of assistance, but that a considerable percentage would. Betty explains:

They should be allowed to stay in hospital a bit longer, until the breastfeeding is established, they've learnt how to settle their babies, just basic little parenting skills, which no-one else is going to be able to teach them we can describe all we want in a one to one situation, but some of them need to be shown by example, you know what I mean, hence the rise of the 'Sleep centres' and the lactation consultants and all the rest of it, I just feel they're coming out with too little skills ...

Mary (M&CHN) suggests that additional assistance was often required by older mothers in order

to master 'ordinary' care:

> *I've got one girl at the moment, who is in this age group and she has no idea what to do,
> she was relying on her husband to do it all and she was heading for postnatal depression,
> so I had to then get her to South Eastern [mother and baby unit], just for a day stay, all she
> needed was a bit of a help with parenting skills, just settling, mother craft type of things,
> just mechanical things ...*

In brief, findings of requiring additional assistance with breastfeeding and 'ordinary' care of the infant

are described almost unanimously by the midwives and M&CHNs and are discussed further in chapter

8.

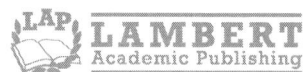
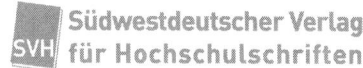

Printed in Great Britain
by Amazon.co.uk, Ltd.,
Marston Gate.